PARTICIPATORY EVALUATION IN YOUTH AND COMMUNITY WORK

Theory and Practice

Susan Cooper

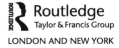

Routledge
Taylor & Francis Group

LONDON AND NEW YORK

First published 2018
by Routledge
2 Park Square, Milton Park, Abingdon, Oxon OX14 4RN

and by Routledge
711 Third Avenue, New York, NY 10017

Routledge is an imprint of the Taylor & Francis Group, an informa business

British Library Cataloguing in Publication Data
A catalogue record for this book is available from the British Library

Library of Congress Cataloging in Publication Data
Names: Cooper, Susan, 1962- author.
Title: Participatory evaluation in youth and community work : theory
    and practice / Susan Cooper.
Description: 1st Edition. | New York : Routledge, 2018. |
    Includes bibliographical references and index.
Identifiers: LCCN 2017037278| ISBN 9781138184374 (hardback) |
    ISBN 9781138184381 (pbk.) | ISBN 9781315645247 (ebook)
Subjects: LCSH: Social work with youth. | Community-based social
    services.
Classification: LCC HV1421 .C66 2018 | DDC 362.7/2532--dc23
LC record available at https://lccn.loc.gov/2017037278

ISBN: 978-1-138-18437-4 (hbk)
ISBN: 978-1-138-18438-1 (pbk)
ISBN: 978-1-315-64524-7 (ebk)

Typeset in Bembo
by Servis Filmsetting Ltd, Stockport, Cheshire

CONTENTS

LIST OF FIGURES

LIST OF TABLES

ACKNOWLEDGEMENTS

The content of this book has been informed by the many and varied experiences I have had throughout my youth and community work career. I would like to offer thanks to all those involved in helping to shape my thinking about evaluation. This includes numerous young people, youth workers and academic colleagues. In particular, I would like to express my thanks to Anu Gretschel for her constructive comments, and for broadening my views, and to my wife Helen Toll for her continued support and encouragement throughout.

INTRODUCTION

This book examines the theory and practice of evaluation in the context of youth and community work, bringing together these two bodies of knowledge in a single text for the first time. It provides the reader with a comprehensive and critical understanding of the intersection between evaluation and youth and community work practice. The complexities of 'evaluating in practice' are explored and the challenges of evidencing the difference that youth and community work makes to the lives of young people and communities are highlighted and examined.

The current appetite for evidence-based practice and the resurgence of the experimental paradigm globally present further challenges to those trying to develop more democratic forms of evaluation. This book offers a timely and unique insight into the use of participatory evaluation for those working with young people. It seeks to raise awareness of the ways in which evaluative practices can shape and be shaped by our understanding of youth work. Critical questions are raised in relation to contemporary forms of evaluation, and alternative paradigms that are more participatory in nature and more akin to the practice of youth and community work are explored. The theory and practice of participatory evaluation is applied to the field of youth and community work, providing the reader with a critical and comprehensive understanding as well as guidance for implementation.

Evaluation is seen as an essential aspect of profession practice. In the UK, for example, students studying to become professional youth workers are explicitly required to involve and support young people in evaluating the impact of youth work activities. However, there is little in terms of current literature to help them achieve this. This book is an essential text for students of all levels preparing for a career in youth and community work, social work and youth development work. It is a valuable resource for students on evaluation and applied evaluation programmes. Youth and community work professionals and professionals in allied fields wanting to improve their evaluation knowledge and practice will also find this a useful resource and guide.

What is youth work?

This book is aimed at those involved in youth and community work. They may be practitioners, students, leaders or academics; all will be committed to working with young people, but the ways in which they understand, articulate and deliver that work may differ. Currently, while there is no universally agreed definition of the term 'youth work', national definitive statements, however, do show common features.

English context

Youth work is informed by a set of beliefs which include a commitment to equal opportunity, to young people as partners in learning and decision-making and to helping young people to develop their own sets of values. The National Youth Agency identifies the following qualities of youth work.

Youth work:

- offers its services in places where young people can choose to participate,
- encourages young people to be critical in their responses to their own experience and to the world around them,
- works with young people to help them make informed choices about their personal responsibilities within their communities,
- works alongside school and college-based education to encourage young people to achieve and fulfil their potential,
- works with other agencies to encourage society to be responsive to young people's needs.

(Ethical Conduct in Youth Work: A statement of values
and principles from the National Youth Agency 2000)

European context

A strategic partnership of nine countries produced a Declaration of Principles of Professional Open Youth Work to serve as a reference point for youth work in Europe.

Professional Open Youth Work:

- creates a safe space where young people can experiment, associate, meet peers and grow as an individual in a positive and supportive environment,
- provides experiences and activities that foster the acquisition of new skills and competencies, broaden horizons and contribute to their personal development,

- creates a stable, respectful and meaningful relationship, based on dialogue and complementary to other relationships such as family, friends, school and work,
- creates opportunities for young people to make positive experiences and supports their participation in their local community and the wider society for empowering them,
- raises the social and (inter-) cultural skills and competencies of young people and thus fosters their inclusion in society,
- applies an holistic approach in all its interactions with young people and supports them during periods of transition, especially during their adolescent years,
- reaches out to all young people including those not actively attending youth work,
- offers and fosters good relations with all other groups present in the community.
  (POWYE Declaration of Principles 2016: 21)

Australian context

Youth work provision in Australia differs from state to state; however, the Australian Youth Affairs Coalition developed a national definition in 2013:

> Youth work is a practice that places young people and their interests first. Youth work is a relational practice, where the youth worker operates alongside the young person in their context. Youth work is an empowering practice that advocates for and facilitates a young person's independence, participation in society, connectedness and realisation of their rights. (Australian Youth Affairs Coalition: National Definition of Youth Work 2013)

USA context

Youth work in the USA is not easily or clearly defined (Velure Roholt and Rana 2011); the term Positive Youth Development (PYD) has become popular in describing work with young people. PYD can be seen as 'asset-based' as it rejects a deficit framing of young people (Schulman and Davies 2007: 4). Its underlying principles are that programmes:

- are universal,
- are strengths-based,
- are structured,
- link process,
- link environment to outcomes. (Schulman and Davies 2007: 4–5)

The PYD process rests on the development of reciprocal relationships between young people and adults in a range of different contexts and environments and the anticipated outcomes can be grouped under five developmental areas: physical, intellectual, psychological, emotional and social. PYD can be seen as an holistic approach as it brings together the biological, psychological and the social, but arguably, this results in a focus on individual development rather than collective learning.

Therefore the answer to the question 'What is youth work?' is not straightforward. There is no unified definition of youth work that applies across Europe or the wider world. Youth work has been informed by distinct national traditions and practices, and consequently variation exists. There are, however, enough common features to allow a shared understanding of its essential nature and to outline its values and outcomes. These common features are:

- **The work must build from where young people are**. The young person's life experience is respected and forms the basis for shaping the agenda in negotiation with peers and youth workers.
- **The relationship between the young person and youth worker is central** to the learning process.
- **Young people and youth workers are active partners in a learning process**. Youth work is a strengths-based approach and holds the belief that young people have strengths and resources. It is these unique strengths and capabilities that will determine their evolving story, not their limitations.
- **It engages with young people within their communities** and acknowledges the wider networks of peers, community and culture.

What are youth work outcomes?

Defining the outcomes of youth work has been troubling the profession for many years. For example, the 2004 study by Bryan Merton et al. concluded that the sector needed to get better at describing, measuring and making the case for the benefits of youth work. There are multiple challenges in defining youth work outcomes. Youth work is a relational practice that is both holistic and emergent (Fusco et al. 2013), and at its core is uncertainty and unpredictability (Ord 2016). There is no established universal starting point from which to establish 'distance travelled', no universal finish line to identify outcomes achieved. Youth work responds to situations that are present in the everyday lives of young people in different contexts. It works in partnership with young people and this cooperative methodology means that outcomes are difficult to predict and difficult to measure (Coburn and Gormally 2014).

For some engaged in youth work, the reluctance to embrace the idea of outcomes is due to scepticism about what could and would be measured. At the root of this is the fear that any attempt to link process to outcome will pave the way for the introduction of universal metrics and experimental evaluation methods that are at odds with the humanist rhetoric of traditional youth work. It is relatively easy to count simple input and output measures, but the challenge is in greater measuring of the nuanced outcomes. A further argument against the introduction of universal outcomes is that it risks undermining the very nature of youth work. Prescribing or predicting outcomes is felt to run counter to the creative and negotiated nature of youth work.

In England, the House of Commons Education Committee (2011) acknowledged in its report that the outcomes of individual youth work relationships are complex and hard to quantify and called for a robust outcome measurement framework to be introduced. The Young Foundation was commissioned to develop this. The resultant Framework for Outcomes for Young People (McNeil, Reeder and Rich 2012) makes the distinction between intrinsic and extrinsic outcomes. Intrinsic outcomes relate to individuals; for example, happiness, self-esteem and confidence, whereas extrinsic outcomes hold a wider benefit; for example, educational achievement, literacy and numeracy or good health. Importantly, it was acknowledged that extrinsic and intrinsic outcomes are often connected and that extrinsic outcomes are easier to measure than intrinsic ones (see Chapter 1 for further discussion). Stuart, Maynard and Rouncefield (2015) use the terms 'proximal' and 'distal' in their discussion on youth work outcomes. Proximal outcomes describe young people's personal development, for example, improvements in their communication or their ability to manage feelings, which results from their engagement in youth work. Distal outcomes relate to longer-term impacts, for example, educational achievement, employment and pro-social behaviour that may result as a consequence of the achievement of proximal outcomes.

Both of these attempts to articulate youth and community work outcomes may support youth workers to identify and communicate the impact of youth work. However, arguably, neither really takes account of the social justice aims of youth work. Collective learning is missing because outcomes are framed through an individual lens. Coburn and Gormally (2014: 70) argue that 'youth work is often caught between an inclination towards a political stance that challenges the status quo and one that is compliant with the prevailing social discourses'. There is a real risk that individualised outcomes that focus on capabilities such as those presented above will tip the balance towards compliance. If youth work is to achieve its social justice aim of encouraging young people to understand and question issues of justice and injustice, of oppression and discrimination, of equity and fairness, then any discussion of outcomes must reflect this.

The lack of clarity about what youth work is may mean that a clear definition of what good practice entails is difficult to ascertain (Velure Roholt and Rana 2011), however, Ord (2016) is keen to point out that the recording of outcomes is not, in itself problematic. He argues that 'The extent to which the recording of outcomes is problematic is dependent on the degree to which they are specifically planned for' (Ord 2016: 154). The push towards prescribing outcomes in order to assess practice against them risks changing the nature of youth work practice. Fusco et al. (2013) support this position arguing that 'youth work is not a one-size-fits-all mould for meeting "targets"'.

However, it is essential that youth work engages with the outcomes discourse, it is no longer an option to insist that youth work outcomes are too complex or too random to be articulated through outcomes. This is not the stance taken by the majority of youth workers who continue to struggle to find ways to articulate the value of their work to a wider audience. The problem rests with the way we conceive outcomes and the measurement of outcomes. The question to be addressed is how can practitioners best make 'value' and 'worth' judgements about the outcomes of their work. Considerable attention has been paid, in England and elsewhere, to developing evaluation frameworks; however, advances have been technical in their nature, rather than political. If the aim is to develop understanding of 'what works and how' so that we are more capable of articulating the value of youth work, we need to critically consider the ways in which evaluation practices enable or disenable us to do this. The aim of this book is to offer an alternative approach to evaluating youth and community work that is more akin to youth work values and practice, through which youth workers and young people can together identify and communicate the value of youth work.

Overview of the book

This book is presented in three parts:

Part 1 explores the dynamic and evolving nature of evaluation. It highlights the dominant discourse and the challenges of these for personnel involved in evaluating youth and community work. It provides underpinning knowledge of the origins, purpose and functions of evaluation and charts the developments in evaluation thinking over the past 50 years. Concepts such as impact, impact measurement and shared measurement are critically examined to illustrate the political nature of evaluation. Findings from empirical research are used to illuminate the tensions and dilemmas that arise from the use of quasi-experimental evaluation in youth and community work.

Part 2 introduces the reader to participatory evaluation and presents an overview of the histories, rationale and underpinning principles. Empowerment evaluation, collaborative evaluation and democratic evaluation are examined in detail, and examples from practice are included to illustrate how these forms of evaluation can be used. Transformative Evaluation, a participatory approach specifically designed for youth and community work is presented. The learning potential associated with participatory forms of evaluation is highlighted.

Part 3 is practice-focused and attention is given to the 'doing' of participatory evaluation. This part of the book offers both a critical examination and guidance to support those new to participatory evaluation in youth and community work. This part of the book will provide a helpful checklist for those already engaging. It provides valuable information on planning, methods, data and data analysis and processes for sharing knowledge.

The concluding chapter returns to the aim of the book which is to promote a re-thinking about how to evidence the difference that youth and community work makes to the lives of young people and communities. The chapter draws together the principles and values of participatory evaluation and youth and community work. It highlights the similarities between the skill sets of participatory evaluators and youth and community workers, concluding with the proposition that youth and community work professionals need to critically question the ways in which their evaluation practice enables or disenables them to develop and communicate the impact and value of youth and community work.

Evaluation is an essential part of professional practice, and the aim of this book is to support students and practitioners, particularly those who have become disengaged from the evaluation process, to recognise the importance and value of their active participation. It is hoped that reading this book will encourage you to embrace the potential of participatory evaluation to develop your ability to more effectively demonstrate and articulate the value of youth and community work to young people, communities, funders and policy-makers.

References

Australian Youth Affairs Coalition (2013) National Definition of Youth Work, accessed at www.youthworkwa.org.au/what-is-youth-work/ (06.07.17)

Coburn, A. and Gormally, S. (2014) 'Emancipatory Praxis: A Social-Justice Approach to Equality Work', in C. Cooper, S. Gormally and G. Hughes (eds), *Socially Just, Radical Alternatives for Education and Youth Work Practice*, Basingstoke: Palgrave Macmillan, pp. 65–84

Fusco, D., Lawrence, A., Matloff-Nieves, S. and Ramos, E. (2013) 'The Accordion Effect: Is Quality in Afterschool Getting the Squeeze?', in *Journal of Youth Development*, Vol. 8(2), accessed at http://jyd.pitt.edu/ojs/jyd/article/view/92 (20.12.16)

House of Commons Education Committee (2011) Services for Young People: Third Report of Session 2010–12, London: The Stationery Office Limited, accessed at www.publications.parliament.uk/pa/cm201012/cmselect/cmeduc/744/744i.pdf (25.08.17)

McNeil, B., Reeder, N. and Rich, J. (2012) A Framework of Outcomes for Young People, accessed at http://youngfoundation.org/wp-content/uploads/2012/10/Framework-of-outcomes-for-young-people-July-2012.pdf (15.04.15)

Merton, B., et al. (2004) *An Evaluation of the Impact of Youth Work in England Research Report RR606*, Nottingham: DfES

NYA (2000) Ethical Conduct in Youth Work: A statement of values and principles from the National Youth Agency, accessed at www.nya.org.uk/wp-content/uploads/2014/06/Ethical_conduct_in_Youth-Work.pdf (21.12.16)

Ord, J. (2016) *Youth Work Process, Product and Practice* (2nd ed.), Oxon: Routledge

Professional Open Youth Work in Europe (POYWE) (2016) Declaration of Principles, accessed at http://poywe.org/site/wp-content/uploads/2016/09/Declaration-of-Principles_Professional-Open-Youth-Work.pdf (06.06.17)

Schulman, S. and Davies, T. (2007) *Evidence of the Impact of the 'Youth Development Model' on Outcomes for Young People: A Literature Review*, Leicester: National Youth Agency

Stuart, K., Maynard, L. and Rouncefield, C. (2015) *Evaluation Practice for Projects with Young People*, London: Sage

Velure Roholt, R. and Rana, S. (2011) 'Improving Community-Based Youth Work: Evaluation of an Action Research Approach', in *Child & Youth Services*, Vol. 32(4), pp. 317–335

PART 1

Evaluation: Nature, politics and tensions

Evaluation is not a universal entity: conceptions of evaluation are socially constructed and thus shaped by a range of economic, political and cultural influences. This part of the book seeks to promote a critical understanding of evaluation through an exploration of its dynamic and evolving nature. The dominant discourse of evaluation is examined and challenged in relation to its use in supporting those engaged in evaluating youth and community work. Whilst much of the content of this part of the book may well be new to many youth and community workers, developing a critical understanding of evaluation is essential to making the case for a more diverse approach to evaluating youth and community work practice.

Chapter 1 ('What is evaluation?') focuses on the evolving nature of evaluation and provides underpinning knowledge of the origins, purpose and functions of evaluation. It charts the developments in evaluation thinking over the past 50 years drawing on a broad range of research (in the UK and internationally) and acknowledges that these developments are influenced by cultural and social forces. The 'Theory of Change' approach is introduced and examined. The chapter concludes with a critical appraisal of evaluation underpinned by the experimental paradigm which is now dominant in many contexts.

Evaluation is inherently political and thus Chapter 2 ('The politics of evaluation') focuses on the impact of neo-liberalism and managerialism on the processes and practices of evaluation in youth and community work. The chapter critically examines the concepts of impact, impact measurement and shared measurement, before examining the 'politics of evidence' through a questioning of what counts as good or credible evidence. Three sets of standards (the 'What Works' Standards, the Nesta Standards and the Bond Principles) are critically reviewed in relation to their applicability in the context of youth and community work evaluation.

The final chapter in this part of the book, Chapter 3 ('Practitioners' tensions and dilemmas') draws on empirical research with youth workers in England. It seeks to illuminate the challenges they experienced as a consequence of using an accountability-focused evaluation. In particular, this chapter examines the value dilemmas they encountered, and the impact they felt the process had on their daily practice.

1

WHAT IS EVALUATION?

This chapter begins by unpacking 'evaluation' in order to consider some of the associated terms such as merit and worth, quality, value and significance. These are explored as a means of establishing a critical awareness of their subjective nature. Paradigmatic approaches influence the way in which we conceive of and practice evaluation; two approaches (positivism and interpretivism) are explored. The dynamic and evolving nature of evaluation in professional practice is then examined in detail. 'Theory of Change' as a basis for evaluation of social programmes has grown in popularity over the past decade. Its origins and developments are examined and its use in relation to youth and community work is explored. Evaluation can be experienced in a variety of ways depending on how it is conceptualised and enacted, and the chapter concludes by offering a critical overview of these responses.

Unpacking 'evaluation'

At a basic level, evaluation can be understood as an everyday activity; we constantly evaluate our experiences, make judgements about the 'value' of the products we use, the relationships we form and the usefulness of our actions. We do this consciously and, more often, subconsciously. Our judgements are subjective, influenced by our values, expectations and our lived experience. However, evaluation, as a professional activity or discipline, is more than this in that while it involves these everyday judgements about value and worth, it entails a much more systematic and rigorous approach. Evaluation in professional contexts is defined in the *Encyclopaedia of Evaluation* as an applied inquiry process for generating and analysing evidence in order to draw conclusions about the value, merit, worth, significance or quality of a programme, product, policy or plan (Fournier cited in Mathison 2005). These terms: 'value', 'merit', 'worth', 'significance' and 'quality' warrant some discussion.

Lincoln and Guba (1986 cited in Mark, Greene and Shaw 2006) make the distinction between merit and worth based on context. They define 'merit' as the intrinsic, context-free qualities of the subject being evaluated. 'Worth' is defined as the context-determined value of the subject being evaluated, in other words, the value of a particular intervention in a particular setting. 'Quality', on the other hand, is an elusive concept (Harvey and Green 1993). Dahlberg, Moss and Pence (2007: 4) problematise the objectification of quality; they argue that 'the concept itself has achieved such dominance that it is hardly questioned. For most part it is taken for granted that there is something – objective, real, knowable – called quality'. Bush and Phillips (1996) support the view that quality needs to be recognised as a social construction as the way in which quality is understood will vary across the world according to the particular stakeholder, their socioeconomic status and culture. They view quality as both a dynamic and relative concept that is subject to change as a variety of factors evolve.

Kelemen (2003) offers two opposing perspectives of quality; the managerial perspective and the critical perspective. The managerial perspective views quality as a technical, operational achievement, seeing it as a self-contained entity that can be planned and controlled with technical and managerial knowledge. This perspective assumes quality can be assessed in a neutral, value-free way through an objective lens. In contrast, the critical perspective views quality as a political, cultural and social concept. This perspective regards quality as a complex and contested social and political phenomenon, which acquires its meaning through processes of communication in which organisational and societal power play a substantial role. The critical perspective argues that quality cannot be studied in a neutral, value-free way through an objective lens.

Conceptions of 'value' and 'significance' are equally evasive, and raise questions as to why greater value or significance is given to one form of outcome as opposed to another. It is necessary to recognise that judgements of value will be informed by how we understand the concept of 'value' and to accept that understanding is contingent and variable. In other words, judgements of 'quality' will be based on subjective conceptualisations of what 'good' practice is and what we believe constitutes 'success' (Mark et al. 2006). What this means then is that different people will have different ways of conceptualising good practice, for example a funder, a senior officer, a practitioner or a service user may all hold different ideas about what quality means.

Weiss (1998: 4) offers a definition of evaluation that takes us forward as it introduces the idea of a set of standards to inform our judgement-making, she states:

> Evaluation is the *systematic assessment* of the *operation* and/or the *outcomes* of a programme or policy, compared to a set of *explicit* or *implicit standards* as a means of contributing to the *improvement* of the policy or programme. (Original emphasis)

It is important to note that in this definition, the standards against which judgements are made can be explicit or implicit. In other words, we must recognise that in the absence of an explicit set of standards, our judgement-making will still be informed by a range of 'markers'. Our 'implicit' standards will be informed by our subjective understanding of 'value' and only be available to us, though not always consciously. By trying to make these 'markers' explicit through dialogue, we can at least surface some of the subjectivities. This is not an easy process as articulating our subjective understanding to others is challenging. People are generally able to recognise quality when they see it, but will struggle to actually define it (Stephenson 2003 cited in McMillan and Parker 2005: 153). However, having an explicit set of standards does not fully address the issue either as these will be subject to interpretation and are likely to be interpreted differently by different people as they draw on their own set of contending influences that are informed by cultural and personal circumstances (Orr 2008).

What is evaluation for?

There is not a single definitive purpose for evalaution but there are some commonalities. Chelminsky (1997) proposes that evaluation has three purposes:

- accountability, which responds to the demands of funders and stakeholders to meet contractual agreements;
- programme development, which focuses on improving the quality of the programme;
- generating knowledge, which aims to develop understanding about what forms of practice are successful.

Everitt and Hardiker (1996) assert that the purpose of evaluation in the context of social welfare should be to promote 'good' practice and firmly situate evaluation in democratic processes. For them, the twin purposes of evaluation involve the generation of evidence about an activity, policy, programme or project and the process of making judgements about its value (Everitt and Hardiker 1996).

Kushner (2000) argues for a different purpose, he makes the connection between evaluation and social justice. For him, evaluation can be a form of political action as it can be used to expose political and intellectual authority. 'Evaluation as political action does not confront society's projects, but it does confront the political infrastructure within which they are designed and operated' (Kushner 2000: 38). Stake (2004) recognises the accountability function of evaluation, but offers a typology of six other functions which he sees as dominant in the context of educational and social programmes:

- assessing goal attainment;
- aiding organisational development;
- assessing contextual quality;
- studying policy aiding social action;
- legitimating the program; and
- deflecting criticism. (Stake 2004: 32)

Taking a critical perspective, there are those who suggest that evaluation can be a technology of control. For example, Trinder's (2000) feminist critique argues that evaluation processes in the context of evidence-based practice can be seen as a covert method of rationing resources and constraining professional autonomy. Davies (2003) supports this view, arguing that evaluation can be regarded both as a product of managerialism and a means of implementing managerialist agendas. Both of these examples relate to forms of evaluation which privilege the accountability function and Issitt and Spence (2005) argue that when evaluation loses its ability to support programme development or generate knowledge it has had a detrimental effect on practice. Dahlberg et al. (2007) argue that evaluation can take on a policing function, positioning it as an integral part of a control system. It is clear then, that while the purpose of any particular evaluation will shape the evaluation approach, it is also important to critically examine the purpose by raising fundamental questions such as what is it we want to know? Why do we want to know this? Who has defined 'quality' and 'value'?

Different paradigmatic approaches

Evaluation is a process of inquiry, it seeks to generate knowledge, and thus evaluation is shaped by the way in which knowledge and knowledge creation is understood. These understandings form our inquiry 'paradigm', that is, the basic set of beliefs that guide our actions. Denzin and Lincoln (2005) provide a thorough account of the various paradigms; here we will briefly consider two: positivism and interpretivism.

Positivism is based on the belief in the ability of scientific knowledge to solve major practical problems (Carr and Kemmis 1986) and is underpinned by an assumption that scientific knowledge is both accurate and certain (Crotty 1998). The positivist paradigm views knowledge as objective and value-free, and therefore generalisable and replicable (Wellington 2000). Evaluation approaches shaped by a positivist paradigm aim to provide explanation and often, although not always, will utilise quantitative methods. Evaluation informed by positivism is generally termed 'experimental' or 'quasi-experimental'. Positivism has its critics; for example, some consider it inappropriate for researching complex social issues (Pring 2000; Whitehead and McNiff 2006) while others, for example Siraj-Blatchford (1994) and O'Donoghue (2007) highlight the lack of recognition and consideration of values as the main problem.

Interpretivism emerged as a reaction to positivism. The interpretive paradigm aims to understand rather than to explain the meaning behind something. It seeks to explore multiple perspectives and develop shared meanings. There are four main assumptions that underpin the interpretive paradigm. These are that:

* knowledge is always situated;
* people construct their 'lived' reality by attaching specific meanings to their experience;

- there is always some degree of autonomy; and
- research involves interaction and negotiation. (O'Donoghue 2007)

The interpretive paradigm assumes that there is no 'one' reality, but instead, there are multiple constructed realities (Denzin and Lincoln 2005) and thus knowledge is subjective and transactional. As such, evaluations informed by an interpretivist paradigm tend towards qualitative methods that create opportunities for accessing multiple voices and perspectives, for example interviews, focus groups and diaries. It is important to note, however, that mixed methods (quantitative and qualitative) are regularly seen. Critics of interpretivism often raise concerns relating to issues of validity, reliability and generalisability. However, arguably these criteria are clearly informed by positivist-inspired aspirations (O'Donoghue 2007). Additionally, critics have questioned the value of inquiry that seeks to describe and understand, arguing that this does not in itself bring about change or challenge the status quo (Carr and Kemmis 1986; Crotty 1988).

In practice, these two paradigms (positivism and interpretivism) are often seen as polar opposites. Positivism is associated with quasi-experimental evaluation approaches which aim to generate information about changes that are measurable, reliable and secure. Interpretivism is associated with the identification and generation of qualitative knowledge with a focus on learning and context.

It is argued elsewhere that the interpretivist paradigm is a more appropriate choice than the positivist paradigm for evaluating youth and community work for two reasons; transparency of values and participation (Cooper 2012). The positivist paradigm claims to be objective and value-free and yet is this really possible? Is it not the case that the subjectivity of the evaluator is simply hidden or ignored? The interpretivist paradigm accepts that the observer makes a difference to what is observed. This acceptance highlights the need for reflexivity; the interpretivist evaluator must explore the ways in which their involvement influences, acts upon and informs their findings. In relation to participation, the interpretivist paradigm supports a more democratic and political approach to evaluation in that it enables us to raise questions about who defines and measures change and for whose benefit this is done (Estrella 2000). Additionally, it prompts us to be open and explicit about the politics, values, and normative aspect of our practice (Abma 2006). Because interpretivism is based on a view of knowledge as 'multiple constructed realities', evaluators informed by this paradigm seek to raise the voices of young people, the community and practitioners in the evaluation process. This focus on participation is contingent with the participatory underpinnings of youth and community work.

In contrast, quasi-experimental evaluations informed by the positivist paradigm seek to identify what works by examining the impact of an intervention, usually by means of measurements before (pre-test) and after (post-test) implementation. This may also involve comparing outcomes for individuals receiving programme activities with outcomes for a similar group of individuals not receiving these activities. While it is accepted that quasi-experimental evaluations of social and educational programs cannot prove that the intervention caused the outcomes (causality), they can produce a range of valuable information, for example about populations served, the achievement of pre-determined outcomes or the magnitude of change. However, quasi-experimental evaluations are criticised on the basis that they often exclude many of the contextual factors that influence cause-and-effect relationships. It is important to acknowledge, however, that our paradigm choice does not necessarily limit our methods of inquiry. Patton (2008) makes the point that paradigm debates go beyond methodology, and argues for a pragmatic approach which recognises and respects difference without trying to reconcile it, and which focuses on the needs of the evaluation.

The evolving nature of evaluation

Approaches to evaluation have changed over time; these changes have been influenced by the rise and fall in the popularity of any particular paradigm. A number of authors have usefully reviewed these changes. Guba and Lincoln (1989) use the concept of four generations of evaluation thinking to illustrate the evolving nature of evaluation. The first of these they termed *the measurement generation* highlighting the critiques of this positivist approach. It was argued that this generation did not address the complex nature of education and social welfare, that the resultant over-simplification was reductionist, relied on a number of quantifiable criteria and falsely claimed validity through measurement. The second generation which they called *the descriptive generation*, focused on the means of achieving desirable outcomes. This generation of thinking attempted to develop understanding of how interventions brought about change. Descriptive understandings can be seen as associated with the interpretive paradigm. The weakness of this generation was seen in the fact that it provided little or no judgement on the value of the processes under study. The third generation, *the judgement generation*, evolved in response to critique of the previous generation. Evaluators began to make judgements claiming that their external position enabled them to be objective. This claim of objectivity can be seen as a return to positivist ideals. *Fourth generation evaluation* dismissed the idea of objective judgement and instead adopted a relative epistemology and a return to the interpretive stance.

Vedung (2010), writing about the major evolutionary trends of evaluation in Sweden, uses a 'wave' metaphor to describe the changing nature of evaluation. In a similar way to Guba and Lincoln (1989) he identifies four cycles or to use his term 'waves' which he suggests have all shaped the way in which we view evaluation today. The wave metaphor is useful as it implies a dynamic rather than static state in relation to thinking about paradigms.

> The whole situation can be likened to ocean waves that roar in and subside, roar in and subside. We can therefore speak of evaluation waves that have swept ashore. In subsiding, the waves have not disappeared without trace but have left behind layers of sediment. In due time, the evaluation landscape has come to consist of layers upon layers of sediment. (Vedung 2010: 265)

The *Science-Driven Wave* occurred during the 1960s when evaluative thinking and practice was driven by a belief that evaluation could make government more rational, scientific and grounded in facts. Evaluation during this period was carried out by professional academic researchers. However, trust and confidence in science to solve social problems began to fade in the 1970s and it was felt that evaluation should be more pluralistic. This led to the *Dialogue-Oriented Wave*, which called for paradigmatic change. Evaluations became informed by the interpretive paradigm to meet the need to include a wide range of stakeholders, including practitioners, service-users and their families. This approach to evaluation was often called 'democratic evaluation'. The 1990s saw a growing dissatisfaction with what some people saw as a concept that was 'based too much on biased ideological beliefs, political tactics, pointless bickering, passing fancies and anecdotal knowledge' (Vedung 2010: 270). The *Dialogue-Oriented Wave* was replaced by the *Neo-Liberal Wave* and a return to positivism was seen with more focus on results and less focus on processes. In contrast to the dialogue-oriented wave, the neo-liberal wave was customer-oriented rather than stakeholder-oriented and, during this period, evaluation became explicitly linked with accountability, performance measurement and consumer satisfaction. The fourth evaluation wave arrived in Sweden from about 2000; Vedung terms this the *Evidence Wave*. This saw a return to experimentation as evaluation focus was firmly on the premise "What matters is what works'. And what works is called evidence' (Vedung 2010: 273). Evidence was ranked on the basis of an evidence hierarchy, with randomised controlled trials and quasi-experimental studies seen as gold standard and qualitative case studies as descriptive examples of good practice. Professional and expert opinion ranked lower and user opinion ranked as the lowest.

Shadish, Cook and Leviton (1991) developed a three-stage model to chart the histories of evaluation theories as shown in Table 1.1.

At the time, this classification model was welcomed as it provided the most comprehensive study of evaluation theory, but as with all models it was criticised by some for what it did not include. Rabie and Cloete (2009) critique the model for its focus on just two variables; rigorous methodologies (associated with scientific principles) and less rigorous methodologies which prioritise use and relevance. They argued that the dynamic nature of evaluation required a new typology to classify the emerging approaches and to make links between classic and contemporary approaches. Their resultant typology identifies three variables for grouping

TABLE 1.1 Three stages of evaluation development (from Shadish, Cook and Leviton 1991)

Stage	Evaluation Focus	Evaluation Approach informed by
Stage I	The discovery of truth	Scientific principles
Stage II	Social utility of evaluation	Use and pragmatism
Stage III	Integration of inquiry and utility	Science and pragmatism

the different evaluation approaches: scope, philosophy and methodology (Rabie and Cloete 2009).

The second of these variables, philosophy, is further explored here. This variable is used to classify evaluation approaches as either theory-driven or participation-driven. Theory-driven evaluations aim to produce in-depth knowledge of the workings of a programme and are based on an implicit 'theory of change' which links activity with intended outcomes. It is important to note that this does not assume a simple linear cause and effect relationship between programme activity and outcomes; rather it recognises the importance and complexity of context and intervention. Participation-driven evaluations, as the term suggests, focus on the engagement of a range of stakeholders with the aim of creating a shared understanding of the programme, its interventions and its outcomes. The level of participation of stakeholders will vary across the many evaluation approaches within this sub-category, but all will be underpinned by a participatory philosophy. Rabie and Cloete's comprehensive work is useful in understanding different evaluation approaches and how they relate to and support each other.

Introducing 'theory of change'

The concept of 'theory of change' began to emerge from 'realistic' evaluation techniques (Pawson and Tilley 1997) in North America during the 1970s and 1980s. This was in response to the need to more effectively take account of context issues and complexity when evaluating social programmes. The term 'theory of change' was coined in the 1990s when the evaluation social enterprise ActKnowledge partnered with the Aspen Institute to establish a practical, theory of change-based evaluation for social programmes. In essence, theory of change can be understood as a theory of how and why an initiative works:

> ... it describes the set of assumptions that explain both the mini-steps that lead to a long term goal and the connections between these activities and the outcomes of an intervention or programme. (Stein and Valters 2012: 5)
>
> ... it is flexible and practical insofar as it clearly articulates a vision of meaningful social change, and then systematically maps out specific steps towards achieving it. (Bours, McGinn and Pringle 2014: 2)

Theory of change emphasises the importance of context in understanding how complex programmes lead to changes in outcomes (Blamey and Mackenzie 2007). Vogel (2012: 4) asserts that theory of change is best seen as 'theory of change thinking'; she argues that it is both a process and a product. The bringing together of outcome data with an understanding of the process that led to those outcomes can enable significant learning about a programme's impact and the enabling factors. Barnett and Gregorowski (2013) identify a key advantage of a theory of change approach is that it can accommodate different views of the change process and provide a mechanism for dialogue between different stakeholder groups. Rogers (2008) points to its value in terms of enabling the articulation of the many underlying assumptions about how change will happen in a programme. It encourages an open dialogue regarding perspectives and values, resulting in a shared vision and stronger relationships with partners and stakeholders. A further benefit of theory of change is that it can be used to bring 'evaluative thinking' into a programme at an early stage.

However, whilst the theory of change approach has proved popular for both evaluators and commissioners of complex social programmes, Mason and Barnes (2007) point out the considerable variation in the ways in which theory of change evaluations have been implemented. It is not a magic bullet; it can be used as poorly or as well as any other approach. There are challenges; for example, it requires a commitment to take a reflective, critical and honest approach to respond to questions about how our efforts might influence change, and this can be difficult given the political realities of the practice environment. The most important criterion for guiding a theory of change evaluation is to be clear about the purpose for which it will be used.

A theory of change approach differs from a 'logic model'. Logic models focus on aligning the component parts of a programme into a hierarchy of clearly-specified goals, objectives, outputs, inputs and activities, often with a set of measurable indicators to demonstrate progress. In contrast, theory of change is broader; it sets out the project 'vision' which is then broken down into a causal pathway with preconditions and assumptions for each step towards that vision. Assumptions, in this context, are statements about how and why we expect the set of outcomes described in a causal pathway to come about, in other words, assumption statements are the 'theories' in theory of change thinking. These statements will reflect understandings of the change process, and may be informed by both research and practical experience. They should also reflect an understanding of the context within which the project operates. The causal pathway is the frame on which all the other details are added. It summarises the theory of change by explaining how the vision (the long-term outcomes) is achieved and describes the preconditions of change at each point. Long-term change is brought about by reaching intermediate preconditions; intermediate change is brought about by reaching early preconditions. In other words, everything on the causal pathway can be understood as a precursor or requirement for the next outcome. Preconditions must be achieved in order for the next step in the sequence to be achieved (see Figure 1.1 for a practice example).

In this example, the long-term goal is to promote pro-social behaviour. To respond to the question of what conditions must exist in order for this outcome to be achieved, the youth project used a backwards mapping process to identify the early stages of the change process. They work on the assumption that increasing involvement and confidence (self and social) can foster young people's competence and sense of achievement. Taking responsibility for self and others through a structured and supported framework, for example, acting as Senior Members enables the internalising of values that underpin and promote pro-social actions. Evaluation is used to identify progress and to develop an understanding of what works at the various stages.

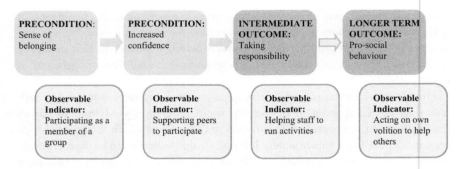

FIGURE 1.1 Outcomes pathway using 'theory of change'

In the last decade the concept of theory of change has grown in popularity in Britain. New Philanthropy Capital (NPC), a UK charity think tank, were commissioned by the Youth Justice Board to deliver theory of change training throughout England and Wales to youth justice practitioners in local authorities and secure establishments. Kail and Lumley (2012) developed guidance for charities in the form of a five-stage process for creating a theory of change (see Table 1.2).

TABLE 1.2 Theory of change: a five-stage process (from Kail and Lumley 2012)

Stage	Action	Description
1	Identify a realistic and definite goal	The goal (programme aim) is the end point of the theory of change. This needs to be stated as clearly as possible and must be achievable otherwise it will be impossible to build a causal model.
2	Work backwards to generate the intermediate outcomes	A backwards mapping process (asking the question 'what has to happen in order for this goal to be achieved?') is used to identify the intermediate outcomes required. This can ensure that the focus is on what has to be done to achieve the goal, rather than on what the current activities are.
3	Establish the links between outcomes, and their order, by working out causes and effects	It is important to examine the links in detail, questioning whether one outcome really leads to the next, and the reasons for believing that.
4	Work out which activities lead to which outcomes	This process of aligning practice to outcomes involves agreeing what needs to be done to achieve the outcomes.
5	Identify what else is needed for the intervention to work	A useful way to approach this stage is to look at what would completely derail the intervention as this can reveal important enabling factors.

Applying theory of change thinking in the context of youth and community work requires us to resolve, or attempt to resolve two conundrums, namely outcomes and causality. There has been much debate about outcomes in youth work over the past two decades. One side of the argument is that outcomes cannot be predetermined as they emerge from the process of youth work (Ord 2016). Others feel that youth work needs to address the challenge of articulating anticipated outcomes. The lack of a common language around youth work outcomes was identified as a barrier. The Outcomes Framework developed by the Young Foundation sought to address this by offering a shared language to assist youth work organisations to articulate and demonstrate the impact of youth work on the lives of young people. The Outcomes Framework distinguishes between intrinsic outcomes and extrinsic outcomes and between individual and social outcomes (see Table 1.3). The interrelated nature of these is acknowledged within the framework.

Theory of change thinking requires a consideration of causality, the second conundrum. Ord (2016) argues that learning (and thus change) results from purposeful activity but does not directly result from a single or a series of specific inputs. Youth work takes place in a 'messy' environment in which numerous different factors interact simultaneously. It is not therefore possible to make claims of causality in a straightforward way. The expectation of funders for proof of causality is a concern across the sector, as is the ability to attribute outcomes to specific intervention (Ellis and Gregory 2008).

Causality can be understood as an hypotheses about how change happens. Pawson and Tilley (1997) use the term 'causal mechanisms' to refer to combinations of context and social processes that an intervention seeks to 'activate'. Other terms have used, for example, 'causal ingredients' (Schorr and Marchand 2007) and 'causal inference' (Funnell and Rogers 2011). Essentially, in theory of change thinking, the aim is to identify the anticipated relationship between the programme's activities and the changes it seeks to bring about. The evaluation design is then shaped to 'test' this theory. This approach to 'causality' does offer new opportunities for

TABLE 1.3 Interrelated outcomes (from the Young Foundation)

Outcome	Description
Intrinsic	Outcomes are primarily valued by individuals and relate to individual well-being, for example, happiness, self-esteem and confidence.
Extrinsic	Outcomes are measurable and valued by other people as well as individuals; examples include educational achievement, literacy and numeracy or good health.
Individual	Outcomes are primarily of interest to the individual and can be both intrinsic and extrinsic, for example, determination, resilience and literacy and numeracy. Individual outcomes contribute to human capital.
Social	Outcomes that impact on society more generally, for example, civic participation and the ability to be a good parent. Social outcomes contribute to social capital.

youth and community workers, and although for some, the conundrums of outcomes and causality will remain, others may find that theory of change thinking can enable a more useful conception of these thorny issues.

In terms of outcomes, the focus is shifted from long-term outcomes to developing a more nuanced understanding of intermediate outcomes, and the inter-relationship between these and long-term outcomes. This allows a 'valuing' of intermediate outcomes which has been absent in the past. Creating causal pathways becomes a collaborative activity in which context and complexity, community and individual resources, knowledge and experience play a part. No longer is causality seen as 'proving the un-provable'.

Theory of change has its critics, for example, some people may find the use of language problematic; the word 'theory' can be viewed as academic and thus exclusionary for those who consider themselves as 'non-academic' (some young people and community members). For others, the idea of identifying 'causal' relationships between intervention and outcome feels too 'mechanistic' to be applied as they conceive youth and community work to be an organic and emergent activity. There is also the question as to whether there is only one 'theory of change'. The evaluation literature on programme theory emphasises that there may be different theories actively influencing a programme.

Drawing on Argyris and Schön's (1974) concept of theories in practice, arguably there is the 'espoused theory' on how a programme 'should' work which is influenced by organisational norms and the 'theory in use' which relates to how a programme is actually implemented. Additionally, different stakeholders may indeed hold different theories of change from those either leading or delivering the programme. These potential differences are not necessarily problematic and supporters of theory of change approaches argue that the process enables these differences to be surfaced and explored. The participatory nature of theory of change means that it is also a time-consuming process. The scope of the process needs to be agreed from the outset, and sufficient resources (time and money) allocated to make sure that it is manageable. Theories of change should help to generate understanding and clarity, be useful in supporting different aspects of the project cycle and be proportionate to the scale of the initiative (Funnell and Rogers 2011).

The problem with evaluation

There is no problem with evaluation per se, the problems arise from the way in which evaluation is conceived and enacted. While evaluation is generally accepted to have three purposes: to determine accountability, to gain new knowledge and to improve agency capability (Chelminsky 1997), it is not a neutral process. It does not take place in a vacuum; it is influenced by current economic, political, historical and social trends (Guba and Lincoln 1989; Vedung 2010). Today evaluation is very much embedded in the culture of accountability (Chouinard 2013), and accountability in the era of managerialism is predominately conceived as technocratic (Greene 1999). In other words, the meaning of accountability has been reshaped from a broad democratic sharing of responsibility (by practitioners to participant, practitioner to self, to professional body, to agency, to funders) to a narrowly-formed conception based on control, regulation and compliance. When evaluation is conceived and enacted as a mechanism for this narrowly framed version of accountability, it becomes problematic for those engaged in youth and community work. Experimental evaluation approaches that are favoured by this version of accountability, objectify individuals and thus are at odds with the core values of youth and community work practice which are participation, empowerment and collaboration.

In summary, evaluation can be experienced in a variety of ways depending on how it is conceptualised and enacted as shown below:

- **As an exclusive or inclusive process:**
  Accountability-focused evaluations are generally externally-driven and are often experienced by practitioners and service users as exclusionary (Issitt and Spence 2005) and predominantly for the benefit of funders and regulators (Ellis and Gregory 2008). Democratic and participatory forms of evaluation are inclusive; they seek to engage as wide a range of stakeholders as possible as active participants in the evaluation process.
- **As controlling or liberating:**
  Evaluation can be experienced as a form of control, both in relation to the control of practitioners and the control of service users. Some forms of evaluation create an upward compliance where the professional is no longer responsible for defining good practice or determining the outcomes of their work. Instead, they are required to produce evidence of externally-set targets. These targets can be seen as form of control in themselves, shaped by normative ideas about what is desirable in societal terms. Conversely, some forms of evaluation can be emancipatory, for example, empowerment evaluation which has a primary objective of helping people to help themselves (Fetterman 1996). Issues of concern are constructed by those involved, as are the means of addressing these concerns and the processes through which success can be ascertained.
- **As a threat or a defense:**
  In the context of performativity, evaluation can be experienced as a threat. The threat arises from concerns that failure to produce 'credible' evidence of worth will be used for punitive purposes or the removal of resources. It is highly risky to admit 'failure' even in those organisations which espouse a commitment to learning from mistakes. In contrast, evaluation can be experienced as an enabling process through which the value of a programme can be identified, articulated, assessed and promoted. Theory of change approaches encourage an open dialogue regarding perspectives and values which can strengthen relationships with partners and stakeholders and engender support for the project.
- **As imposition or as part of everyday professional practice:**
  Some forms of evaluation, particularly those associated with accountability-focused approaches, can be experienced as the imposition of rigorous regimes

of externally managed monitoring and auditing systems. These require practitioners to spend significant time and energy in detailed administration and documentation. When evaluation is reduced to data production, particularly quantitative data which fails to recognise or capture what they consider to be the valuable or important aspects of their work, practitioners are likely to view the process as having limited value for them (Derrick-Mills 2011) and as a distraction from their 'real' work. Alternatively, if the evaluation approach is congruent with the ethos of practice, and when the processes recognise the validity of professionals' 'practice wisdom', practitioners are likely to see how evaluation can both demonstrate the value of their everyday practice and improve their everyday practice. Dialogical and reflective evaluation approaches which support learning and development are more likely to be experienced as an important aspect of professional practice.

References

Abma, T. (2006) 'The Practice and Politics of Responsive Evaluation', in *American Journal of Evaluation*, Vol. 27(1), pp. 31–43

Argyris, C. and Schön, D. (1974) *Theory in Practice: Increasing Professional Effectiveness*, San Francisco: Jossey-Bass

Barnett, C. and Gregorowski, R. (2013) IDS Practice Paper in Brief 14, Brighton: Institute of Development Studies

Blamey, A. and Mackenzie, M. (2007) 'Theories of Change and Realistic Evaluation: Peas in a Pod or Apples and Oranges?' in *Evaluation*, Vol. 13(4), pp. 439–455

Bours, D., McGinn, C. and Pringle, P. (2014) The Theory of Change approach to climate change adaptation programming. SEA Change CoP, Phnom Penh and UKCIP, Oxford, accessed at www.seachangecop.org (02.08.16)

Bush, J. and Phillips, D. (1996) 'International Approaches to Defining Quality', in S. Kagan and N. Cohen (eds), *Reinventing Early Care and Education: A Vision for a Quality System*, San Franciso: Jossey-Bass, pp. 65–80

Carr, W. and Kemmis, S. (1986) *Becoming Critical: Education, Knowledge and Action Research*, London: The Falmer Press

Chelminsky, E. (1997) 'Thoughts for a New Evaluation Society', in *Evaluation*, Vol. 3(1), pp. 97–118

Chouinard, J. (2013) 'The Case for Participatory Evaluation in an Era of Accountability', in *American Journal of Evaluation*, Vol. 34(2), pp. 237–253

Cooper, S. (2012) 'Evaluation: Ensuring Accountability or Improving Practice?', in J. Ord (ed.), *Critical Issues in Youth Work Management*, Abingdon: Routledge, pp. 82–95

Crotty, M. (1998) *The Foundations of Social Research: Meaning and Perspective in the Research Process*, London: Sage Publications

Dahlberg, G., Moss, P. and Pence, A. (2007) *Beyond Quality in Early Childhood Education and Care* (2nd ed.), Abingdon: Routledge

Davies, B. (2003) 'Death to Critique and Dissent? The Policies and Practices of New Managerialism and of "Evidence-based Practice"', in *Gender and Education*, 15(1), pp. 91–103

Denzin, N. and Lincoln, Y. (eds) (2005) *The Sage Handbook of Qualitative Research* (3rd ed.), London: Sage Publications

Derrick-Mills, T. (2011) 'Building the Value of Evaluation: Engaging with Reflective Practitioners', in S. Mathison (ed.), *Really New Directions in Evaluation: Young Evaluators' perspectives,* New Directions for Evaluation, No. 131, pp. 83–90

Ellis, J. and Gregory, T. (2008) *Accountability and Learning: Developing Monitoring and Evaluation in the Third Sector,* London: Charities Evaluation Services

Estrella, M. (2000) 'Learning from Change', in M. Estrella with J. Bluaret, D. Campilan, J. Gaventa, J. Gonsalves, I. Guijt, D. Johnson and R. Ricafort (eds), *Learning From Change: Issues and Experiences in Participatory Monitoring and Evaluation,* London: Intermediate Technology Publications Ltd, pp. 1–13

Everitt, A. and Hardiker, P. (1996) *Evaluating for Good Practice,* Basingstoke: Palgrave

Fetterman, D. (1996) *Empowerment Evaluation: Knowledge and Tools for Self-Assessment & Accountability,* Thousand Oaks, CA: Sage Publications

Funnell, S. and Rogers, P. (2011) *Purposeful Programme Theory: Effective Use of Theories of Change and Logic Models,* San Francisco: Jossey-Bass

Greene, J. (1999) 'The Inequality of Performance Measures', in *Evaluation,* Vol. 5, pp. 160–172

Guba, E. and Lincoln, Y. (1989) *Fourth Generation Evaluation,* London: Sage Publications

Harvey, L. and Green, D. (1993) 'Defining Quality', in *Assessment and Evaluation in Higher Education,* Vol. 18(1), pp. 9–34

Issitt, M. and Spence, J. (2005) 'Practitioner Knowledge and Evidence-based Research, Policy and Practice', in *Youth & Policy,* Vol. 88, pp. 63–82

Kail, A. and Lumley, T. (2012) Theory of Change: The beginning of making a difference, London: New Philanthropy Capital, accessed at www.thinknpc.org/publications/theory-of-change/ (25.08.17)

Kelemen, M. (2003) *Managing Quality: Managerial and Critical Perspectives,* London: Sage Publications

Kushner, S. (2000) *Personalising Evaluation,* London: Sage Publications

Mark, M., Greene, J. and Shaw, I. (2006) 'The Evaluation of Policies, Programs and Practices', in I. Shaw, J. Greene and M. Mark (eds), *The Sage Handbook of Evaluation,* London: Sage Publications, pp. 1–30

Mason, P. and Barnes, M. (2007) 'Constructing Theories of Change: Methods and Sources', *Evaluation,* Vol. 13(2), pp. 151–170

Mathison, S. (ed.) (2005) *Encyclopaedia of Evaluation,* Thousand Oaks, CA: Sage Publications

McMillan, W. and Parker, M. (2005) 'Quality is Bound Up with Our Values: Evaluating the Quality of Mentoring Programmes', in *Quality in Higher Education,* Vol. 11(2), pp. 151–160

O'Donoghue, T. (2007) *Planning Your Qualitative Research Project: An Introduction to Interpretivist Research in Education,* Abingdon: Routledge

Ord, J. (2016) *Youth Work Process, Product and Practice* (2nd ed.), Abingdon: Routledge

Orr, S. (2008) 'Real or Imagined? The Shift from Norm Referencing to Criterion Referencing in Higher Education', in A. Havnes and L. McDowell (eds), *Balancing Dilemmas in Assessment and Learning in Contemporary Practice,* Abingdon: Routledge, pp. 133–143

Patton, M. (2008) *Utilization-focused Evaluation* (4th ed.), London: Sage Publications

Pawson, R. and Tilley, N. (1997) *Realistic Evaluation,* London: Sage Publications

Pring, R. (2000) *Philosophy of Educational Research,* London: Continuum

Rabie, B. and Cloete, F. (2009) 'A New Typology of Monitoring and Evaluation Approaches', in *Administratio Publica,* Vol. 17(3), pp. 76–97

Rogers, P. (2008) 'Using Programme Theory for Complicated and Complex Programmes', in *Evaluation,* Vol. 14(1), pp. 29–48

Schorr, L. and Marchand, V. (2007) Pathway to Children Ready for School and Succeeding at Third Grade, Working Paper, Harvard Pathways Mapping Initiative, Harvard

University, accessed at www.cssp.org/publications/pathways-to-outcomes/3rd-grade-pathway-pdf-9-07.pdf (25.08.17)

Shadish, W., Cook, T. and Leviton, L. (1991) *Foundations of Program Evaluation: Theories of Practice*, Thousand Oaks, CA: Sage Publications

Siraj-Blatchford, I. (1994) *Praxis Makes Perfect: Critical Educational Research for Social Justice*, Derbyshire: Education Now Books

Stake, R. (2004) 'Stake and Responsive Evaluation', in C. Alkin (ed.), *Evaluation Roots, Tracing Theorists' Views and Influences*, Thousand Oaks, CA: Sage Publications

Stein, D. and Valters, C. (2012) *Understanding Theory of Change in International Development*, Justice and Security Research Program and The Asia Foundation, accessed at www.seachangecop.org/node/1303 (02.08.16)

Trinder, L. (ed.) (2000) *Evidence-based Practice: A Critical Appraisal*, Oxford: Blackwell Science Ltd

Vedung, E. (2010) 'Four Waves of Evaluation Diffusion', in *Evaluation*, Vol. 16(3), pp. 263–277

Vogel, I. (2012) Review of the use of 'Theory of Change' in international development, DFID, accessed at www.gov.uk/government/news/dfid-research-review-of-the-use-of-theory-of-change-in-international-development (02.08.16)

Weiss, C. (1998) *Evaluation: Methods for Studying Programs and Policies* (2nd ed.), New York: Prentice Hall

Wellington, J. (2000) *Educational Research: Contemporary Issues and Practical Approaches*, London: Continuum Books

Whitehead, J. and McNiff, J. (2006) *Action Research: Living Theory*, London: Sage Publications

2

THE POLITICS OF EVALUATION

Introduction

Evaluation is inherently political. It is concerned with generating 'knowledge' and thus, as discussed in Chapter 1, evaluation, as a process, is subject to the 'paradigm wars' that affect social science research more broadly. There are different 'ways of knowing' and these are underpinned by relations of power. For example, the questions we ask in order to generate knowledge will be informed by our 'taken for granted understandings and dominant ways of seeing things in a society divided by gender, race, class, sexuality, disability and age' (Shaw and Compton 2003: 202). The practice of evaluation is a political activity, socially constructed and politically articulated. Further, Taylor and Balloch (2005) assert that evaluation is not only informed by but also contributes to political and policy discourses on a range of levels. Notions of value and quality are contested, and the question of 'what works?' may appear neutral but is indeed politically laden.

This chapter begins by exploring the political landscape that has led to the dominance of the experimental paradigm in evaluating work with young people and communities. The applicability of this particular paradigm for evaluating youth and community work needs to be questioned on the basis that it assumes that outcomes can be prescribed and quantified and attributed to particular programme activities. Good evaluation is seen to provide credible and useful evidence; however, perspectives of 'credible' and 'useful' warrant further investigation. Questions need to be raised – what exactly is it that we are trying to evidence? How do we measure success or failure? Who defines 'success' and who decides what constitutes 'credible' evidence? These questions need to be viewed through a critical lens to identify their political nature. The concept of 'shared measurement', which underpins much of the recent developments in evaluation practice in the UK and USA, is explored in this chapter. A range of evidence standards are presented and critiqued.

The political context

In order to understand the dominance of the experimental evaluation paradigm, it is necessary to review the influence of the political context, 'neoliberalism', on the way in which youth and community work organisations are managed. Essentially, neoliberalism favours free-market capitalism and prioritises economy, effectiveness and quality (Rose 2010). Managerialism is a product of neoliberalism, and its aim is to bring about organisational change in order to meet the competitive challenge of a global economy. In other words, managerialism seeks to improve the performance of the public services through the introduction of managerial techniques taken from private enterprise (Clarke and Newman 1997).

Managerialism is characterised by the assessment of quality using external, objective benchmarks generally involving quantitative methods such as performance indicators and externally imposed targets. Arguably, these forms of assessment have undermined the level of trust placed on the professional (O'Neill 2002; Avis 2003) and lead to new forms of organisational control (Clarke 1998). In this political context, evaluation is very much embedded in a culture of accountability (Chouinard 2013), and accountability is predominately perceived as technocratic.

The pressure to demonstrate the effectiveness of youth and community work has, and is continuing to increase. In England, decreasing resources and the need to show 'value for money' were powerful drivers behind the *Transforming Youth Work* (DfES 2002) policy for statutory-funded youth services. *Resourcing Excellent Youth Services* (DfES 2004) introduced externally-set targets for state-funded youth work. For the first time, youth services were evaluated against quantifiable targets for attendance, participation, accredited and recorded outcomes. The inappropriateness of this form of evaluation in youth work was striking. Setting measurable outcomes is quite straightforward when the 'product' is tangible, for example, a Youth Achievement Award or a Duke of Edinburgh Certificate. However, youth work is a qualitative process; it is concerned with developing individuals and groups, with personal and social development and, as such, indentifying outcomes that lend themselves to measurement is problematic. The pressure to set outcomes which were quantifiable led many youth services to focus their attention on those things that are easily counted, for example, contacts or accreditations. These targets had a detrimental effect on youth work practice as essentially they delimited practice and determined outcomes (Spence 2004).

A further example of the growing dominance of the experimental paradigm in the English context was seen in the promotion of 'Outcome Based Accountability' by the Department for Children, Schools and Families (DCSF, now DfE). Outcome Based Accountability (OBA), developed by Friedman (2005) in the USA, was adopted by a number of Children's Trusts. The following extract from the publication *Better Outcomes for Children and Young People – From Talk to Action* is clearly informed by a positivist paradigm;

Work is underway to try to understand what works best in 'narrowing the gap' in outcomes, through the Narrowing the Gap Project. This project, (...) is one of a number of initiatives which aims to understand *what action, if applied universally and pursued relentlessly, would make a significant impact on the outcomes* of vulnerable groups of children and young people. It is seeking *to identify the simple truths rooted in evidence* across all five outcomes that will assist local authorities and their partners to take effective action. (DCSF 2008: 6, author's emphasis)

The language associated with this 'what works?' approach may appear pragmatic and neutral. However, the emphasis on 'common sense' and 'simple truths', particularly in terms of the three 'common sense' performance measures (How much did we do? How well did we do it? and Is anyone better off?) is political. Using terms such as 'common sense' and 'simple' in this way silences any dissenting voices, since how can one argue against common sense? And why is it that one does not understand when it is so simple? The hidden danger of OBA is that the collaboration and participation of users is used to legitimise what remains essentially a managerialist process. To ask a range of stakeholders 'How well did we do?' in a meaningful way requires a paradigm shift, from realist to relativist, from 'one truth' to 'multiple truths', and from positivism to interpretivism because people will have different conceptualisations of quality (Kelemen 2003).

This shift of focus towards seeing evaluation as a key mechanism of the accountability movement can be seen as a cause for concern on three counts. Firstly, it favours an experimental evaluation paradigm, with its associated quasi-scientific methods that rely on pre-defined and universal causal pathways between intervention and outcome. This approach to evaluation is seen as incongruent with youth and community work values and, importantly, it is inadequate for capturing the complexity and demonstrating the value of this work (see Ball 2003). Ling (2012) highlights the challenges of conducting accountability-focused evaluation in contexts where interventions are complex, arguing that complexity makes it difficult to describe in advance what interventions will do or what outcomes might result.

Secondly, the current discourse of accountability has reshaped the meaning of accountability. It is no longer understood as a broad democratic sharing of responsibility (by practitioners to participant, practitioner to self, to professional body, to agency, to funders). Accountability, in the context of managerialism is viewed as a narrowly-formed technocratic conception that is based on control, regulation and compliance. Evaluation is reduced to upward compliance; the professional is no longer responsible for defining good practice or determining the outcomes of their work.

Thirdly, the pressure to demonstrate effectiveness and the dominance of the experimental paradigm has, for many, shifted the focus of evaluation from one of 'improving' programmes to one of 'proving the worth' of programmes. This is potentially damaging the long-term future of youth and community work as issues of process and implementation are missed and our ability to understand the richness and complexity of the work is impeded. Spenceley (2006: 300) asserts that the impact of organisational demands for evidence affects what professionals do, changing their primary focus from the provision of a service to: 'proving the value of the "service" offered through a range of statistical measurements and customer satisfaction surveys, ensuring that the organisational "quality standards" ... are met.'

Clearly, demonstrating the difference that youth and community work makes to the lives of young people and organisational effectiveness are important and valuable but, equally, these are politically-laden concepts. How do we 'measure' effectiveness and impact in the context of youth and community work? It is important to note that things have moved on in relation to this question. There have been concerted efforts to move away from focusing on just those things that are easily quantifiable (generally referred to as outputs, for example, the number of sessions delivered, the number of people attending) to developing a more nuanced understanding of 'impact'. However, the dominant discourse remains one of quantification.

Understanding 'impact'

In a climate of decreasing resources there is, understandably, a greater level of scrutiny of how resources are used. The introduction of 'payment by results' and other procurement mechanisms that aim to ensure scarce resources are directed to programmes that generate the biggest effects may seem both logical and necessary. However, the challenge to provide more and better evidence of impact is considerable. The starting point, surely, is the question of what is it that we are trying to prove, followed by how can we prove this? These are not simply methodological questions, they are political. These foundational questions are answered by those who have the power to influence; who this includes or excludes will be informed by the evaluation purpose, which in turn will influence the evaluation approach and design. Deciding what is to be evaluated and how, is a political act, the way we frame this will depend on dominant social policy and the ways in which social issues are constructed and understood (Pawson and Tilley 1997).

Putting this into context, there are two factors at play in the current policy discourse; the first factor is the individualisation movement which focuses on psychological dispositions rather than structural inequalities. Social problems are addressed on an individual basis; structural constraints are not ignored, but they are seen as obstacles for the individual to overcome. Interventions are targeted at those young people who are deemed not to have the capacity to overcome the barriers they face. The success of the intervention is assessed at an individual level. The second factor is the neoliberal belief in a market economy to achieve the best outcome with the available resource. This premise requires an ability to make comparisons, to be able to judge one project against another. In this scenario, a quasi-experimental evaluation design may be seen as the best way to produce evidence that can be used to make this judgement. Particular methods, for example, control groups and pre-post tests are used to generate objective, quantifiable, and robust data to show that a prescribed causal pathway works. However, how we define success remains a challenge, particularly in relation to the programme comparison element. Attempts have been made to address this challenge through the development of 'shared measurement'.

Shared measurement

In 2012 New Philanthropy Capital conducted a survey to gauge the state of impact measurement across the UK charity sector. They found that while over 50 per cent of the participating charities were measuring impact for all or nearly all of their activities, almost 25 per cent were not measuring impact at all. Their findings suggested a combination of factors were at play which prevented organisations from measuring impact effectively, or in some cases, at all. These included being uncertain as to how to identify outcomes, a lack of availability of appropriate measurement tools, difficulties in analysing results, a lack of funding for impact measurement, and the competing (and often diverse) data demands from funders.

In the same year the Young Foundation published *A Framework of Outcomes for Young People*. The purpose of the framework was clearly stated as:

> not intended as a formal performance management or accountability framework for national or local government. While its development has been funded by the Department for Education, the emphasis is on empowering providers and commissioners to articulate and demonstrate impact in improving outcomes for young people. (McNeil, Reeder and Rich 2012: 2)

A Framework of Outcomes sought to provide a shared language through which youth and community work providers could articulate the difference their work makes to the lives of young people. The framework offers guidance as to how to measure impact based on a set of identified capabilities and includes a number of relevant and useful tools.

The year 2013 saw the publication of the 'Blueprint for Shared Measurement' which, drawing on an analysis of twenty approaches already in operation in the UK and the USA, set out a concept of shared measurement for UK charities and social enterprises. Shared measurement involves bringing together organisations that work on similar issues and similar goals to develop a common understanding of what to measure, and how to develop the tools to do so. Shared measurement is defined as:

> both the product and process of taking a shared approach to impact measurement. In terms of the product, shared measurement is any tool that can be used by more than one organisation to measure impact. The process of shared measurement entails understanding a sector's shared outcomes, often mapping out its theory of change. It also involves the engagement and collaboration needed to result in a shared approach. (Ní Ógáin, Svistak and de Las Casas 2013:6)

The concept of shared measurement has its advantages, particularly in relation to economics; for example, the pooling of expertise and resources to develop measurement practice can save time and money and avoid duplication. It could lead to the rationalisation of funders' data requirements, again saving time and money. Clearly, the economic benefits are likely to be welcomed by organisations that are forever required to do more with less. However, a degree of caution may be necessary as shared measurement also has the potential to be used for comparative purposes, judging one project against another in the competitive marketplace. This potential is perhaps missing from the claim that:

> The ultimate aim of shared measurement is to build information about what works in solving social problems. Having more comparable and robust data on the impact of different programmes can help us identify trends in what leads to positive change across a number of different social issues. (Ní Ógáin, Svistak and de Las Casas 2013: 9)

What counts as 'evidence'?

The requirement for robust and comparable evidence of impact has resulted in the development of a range of different approaches, for example social accounting, social return on investment and cost–benefit analysis. There is also more emphasis on rigorous methods of measurement. In 2013 the Social Research Unit (SRU) developed the 'What Works' Standards of Evidence' for those working with children and young people, in part to address the question of how to compare and contrast the different types of evidence being used by organisations to support their claims of impact. The SRU worked with international partners to develop the standards which focus on four areas and the model uses two ratings, 'good enough' and 'best', to assess the quality of interventions. These standards are:

- **Intervention specificity:**
  This standard focuses on three key aspects; what the intervention is, what the intervention tries to achieve and for whom, and how the intervention is supposed to work – essentially the intervention's theory of change.
- **Evaluation quality:**
  This standard relates to the level of confidence in the evaluation design to produce robust and reliable evidence. Two types of evaluation designs are seen as acceptable; randomised controlled trials and quasi-experimental evaluations. The use of validated measurement instruments and appropriate statistical analysis are seen as crucial elements in the judgement of evaluation quality.
- **Intervention impact**:
  This standard relates to how much difference the intervention makes and requires clear evidence of a positive impact of the intervention on the outcomes for the beneficiary and no evidence of a harmful effect. The use of

'effect size' (an *effect size* is a quantitative measure of the strength of a phenomenon) is encouraged.

- **System readiness**:
  This standard is concerned with whether the intervention can be 'scaled
  up' in relation to whether the organisation has the necessary materials, procedures and support in place. The standard also requires information about
  the financial and human resources required to deliver the intervention
  elsewhere.

These standards are designed to support funders and commissioners to make
decisions about where to invest by identifying 'tried and tested' interventions.
Organisations looking to increase the impact of their work can use the standards as
a self-assessment tool. Additionally, evaluators can use the standards as a guide to
conducting rigorous impact measurements. However, on a cautionary note, while
these standards may support the development of an evidence-base which currently
is lacking, they clearly promote an experimental evaluation approach. The value or
applicability of these standards for small-scale projects or indeed for frontline staff
in their everyday practice, is therefore questionable.

The Nesta Standards of Evidence (Puttick and Ludlow 2013) is informed by the
'What Works' Evidence Standards. Interestingly they claim not to be aligned to
any particular data type or specific methods of generating data. Instead, they declare
their interest is 'in high quality, robust and appropriate evidence which helps identify the most promising innovations' (Puttick and Ludlow 2013: 2). The Nesta
Standards use a five-level scale to indicate the level of 'certainty' that any particular
intervention will have a positive impact as summarised in Table 2.1.

Organisations starting out on the 'impact measurement' journey may find the
developmental aspect of these standards useful and encouraging. What is interesting
in relation to these standards is the assertion that they are paradigm-free. The claim to
not demand particular methods is somewhat incongruent with the inclusion at level 2,
of suggested methods such as pre- and post-survey evaluation, and at level 3, the
use of control groups, random selection and sizeable populations. As with the 'What
Works' standards, the Nesta Standards may provide a useful organisational management resource, but only limited support for small-scale projects and front-line staff.

TABLE 2.1 The Nesta Standards of Evidence (from Puttick and Ludlow 2013: 2)

Level 1	Able to describe what you do and why it matters logically, coherently and convincingly.
Level 2	Able to capture data that shows positive change, but you cannot confirm you caused this.
Level 3	Able to demonstrate causality using a control or comparison group.
Level 4	Able to provide one or more independent replication evaluations that confirms these conclusions.
Level 5	Able to provide manuals, systems and procedures to ensure consistent replication and positive impact.

The Bond Evidence Principles represent a third set of standards, also launched in 2013. Bond is a UK membership body for organisations working in international development united by a common goal to eradicate global poverty. The dual purposes of the Principles are to assess the quality of existing evidence and to act as a guide when thinking about how evidence can be generated. The five principles are as follows:

- *Voice and inclusion*: the perspective of living in poverty, including the most marginalised, are included in the evidence and a clear picture is provided of who is affected and how.
- *Appropriateness*: the evidence is generated using methods that are justifiable given the nature of the purpose of the assessment.
- *Triangulation*: the evidence has been generated using a mix of methods, data sources, and perspectives.
- *Contribution*: the evidence explores how change happens and the contribution of the intervention and factors outside of the intervention in explaining change.
- *Transparency*: the evidence discloses the details of the data sources and methods used, the results achieved, and any limitations in the data or conclusions.

Using a four-point scale, evidence is judged to be weak, minimum standard, good practice or gold standard.

The language used in this set of standards is quite different to that used in the previous two examples. A key difference is seen in the belief that the inclusion of the beneficiaries in the whole evaluation process (from design, through data generation and analysis, to validating the findings) will provide richer and more compelling evidence of impact. Involving multiple voices in the triangulation process is also seen as vital. There is no direct mention of methods associated with quasi-experimental evaluations, rather there is an emphasis on justification of methods used, thus allowing scope for organisations to negotiate context-appropriate methods and potentially, a shared development process.

These standards are clearly informed by Bond's values which include justice and solidarity, diversity and mutual respect, collaboration and participation, sustainability and shared responsibility, and transparency and accountability. These values are shared by many working with young people and communities, and as such, it may be these principles that are most useful in terms of developing thinking about what constitutes credible evidence when evaluating youth and community work. Mertens and Hesse-Biber (2013) support the call for a broader definition of credible evidence and indeed for the use of mixed methods to generate it, arguing that a deeper understanding of what counts as evidence and more diverse ways of generating it, will enable practitioners to more fully capture the impact of their work.

In summary, there are significant risks associated with accepting the dominant discourse of 'what works?' in the evaluation of youth and community work. The political nature of what is sometimes presented as a neutral, values-free process must be understood if youth and community work is to remain true to its ethos and retain its purpose. The development of a 'shared' language needs to be challenged in terms of who creates that language and for what purpose. Developments in terms of impact measurement have been rooted in the experimental paradigm, and this remains problematic.

References

Avis, J. (2003) 'Rethinking Trust in a Performative Culture', in *Journal of Education Policy*, Vol. 18(3), pp. 315–332

Ball, S. (2003) 'The Teacher's Soul and the Terrors of Performativity', in *Journal of Education Policy*, Vol. 18(2), pp. 215–228

Chouinard, J. (2013) 'The Case for Participatory Evaluation in an Era of Accountability', in *American Journal of Evaluation*, Vol. 34(2), pp. 237–253

Clarke, J. (1998) 'Thriving on Chaos? Managerialism and Social Welfare', in J. Carter (ed.), *Post-Modernity and the Fragmentation of Welfare*, London: Routledge

Clarke, J. and Newman, J. (1997) *The Managerial State*, London: Sage Publications

DCSF (2008) *Better Outcomes for Children and Young People – From Talk to Action*, London: DCSF

DfES (2004) *Transforming Youth Work – Resourcing Excellent Youth Services*, London: DfES

DfES (2002) *Transforming Youth Work*, London: DfES/Connexions

Friedman, M. (2005) *Trying Hard is Not Good Enough: How to Produce Measurable Improvements for Customers and Communities*, Oxford: Trafford Publications

Kelemen, M. (2003) *Managing Quality: Managerial and Critical Perspectives*, London: Sage Publications

Ling, T. (2012) 'Evaluating Complex and Unfolding Interventions in Real Time', in *Evaluation*, Vol. 18(1), pp. 79–91

McNeil, B., Reeder, N. and Rich, J. (2012) *A Framework of Outcomes for Young People*, The Young Foundation, accessed at http://youngfoundation.org/wp-content/uploads/2012/10/Framework-of-outcomes-for-young-people-July-2012.pdf (23.02.17)

Mertens, D. and Hesse-Biber, S. (2013) 'Mixed Methods and Credibility of Evidence in Evaluation', *New Directions for Evaluation*, No. 138, pp. 5–13

Ní Ógáin, E., Svistak, M. and de Las Casas, L. (2013) Blueprint for Shared Measurement: Developing, Designing and Implementing Shared Approaches to Impact Measurement, New Philanthropy Capital, accessed at http://inspiringimpact.org/wp-content/uploads/2013/03/blueprint-for-shared-measurement2.pdf?Downloadchecked=true (23.02.17)

O'Neill, O. (2002) *A Question of Trust*, Cambridge: Cambridge University Press

Pawson, R. and Tilley, N. (1997) *Realistic Evaluation*, London: Sage Publications

Puttick, R. and Ludlow, J. (2013) Standards of Evidence: An Approach that Balances the Need for Evidence with Innovation, Nesta, accessed at www.nesta.org.uk/sites/default/files/standards_of_evidence.pdf (23.02.17)

Rose, J. (2010) 'Monitoring and Evaluating Youth Work', in T. Jeffs and M. Smith (eds), *Youth Work Practice*, Basingstoke: Palgrave Macmillan, pp. 156–167

Shaw, I. and Compton, A. (2003) 'Theory, Like Mist on Spectacles, Obscures Vision', in *Evaluation*, Vol. 9(2), pp. 192–204

Spence, J. (2004) 'Targeting, Accountability and Youth Work Practice', in *Practice: A Journal of the British Association of Social Workers*, Vol. 16(4), pp. 261–272

Spenceley, L. (2006) '"Smoke and Mirrors": An Examination of the Concept of

Professionalism within the FE Sector', in *Research in Post-Compulsory Education*, Vol. 11(3), pp. 289–302

Taylor, D. and Balloch, S. (eds) (2005) *The Politics of Evaluation*, Bristol: The Policy Press

Watty, K. (2003) 'When Will Academics Learn About Quality?', in *Quality in Higher Education*, Vol. 9(3), pp. 213–221

3

PRACTITIONERS' TENSIONS AND DILEMMAS

Introduction

The previous chapters have deconstructed evaluation in order to reveal its composition and to expose its political nature. The reasons for the dominant discourse of evaluation as a process based on the identification of measurable inputs, outputs and outcomes have been examined and it has been argued that setting measurable outcomes in advance that lend themselves to measurement, is incongruent with the qualitative nature of youth and community work.

Watson and Emery (2010) assert that social and emotional learning outcomes are both poorly articulated and contestable, adding that programmes aimed at developing young people's social and emotional learning generate far more outcomes than are recorded. Ord (2007) provides an example of this when he discusses confidence as a youth work outcome and Brent (2004) provides another good example of the intangible nature of youth work outcomes when he describes a young woman's journey in from the periphery as she moved from 'a shadowy appendage of her boyfriend' to 'throw[ing] herself into the life of the Centre' (Brent 2004: 70).

In the context of 'what's measured is what matters', youth and community workers face serious challenges in their daily work. They feel alienated from the evaluation process as a result of the incompatibility of the experimental paradigm with the reality of their practice (Everitt and Hardiker 1996). Issitt and Spence (2005) argue that dominant modes of evidence-gathering, which privilege hard data, serve to silence the voice of the practitioner. This argument is supported by Ellis (2009) who reported that practitioners in the voluntary sector predominantly believe that evaluation is for the benefit of funders and regulators. This chapter explores the lived experience of youth and community work practitioners and in doing so identifies the detrimental effects of an over-reliance on the experimental evaluation approach.

The chapter draws on empirical data from a doctoral research project (Cooper 2012) that sought to illuminate the experiences of a small group of youth and community workers in an English voluntary sector youth project. The project received a central government grant aimed at building long-term organisational capacity and the receipt of this funding involved the introduction of a new accountability-focused evaluation process. Six practitioners were interviewed six months after the receipt of the grant and the texts in italics are direct quotations from those interviews. Analysis of data gathered via in-depth semi-structured interviews provides an interesting insight into the everyday tensions and dilemmas that resulted, in particular the external direction of their work and the challenge to their professional values, purpose and ethos.

Generating data replaces 'real' work

The introduction of monitoring and reporting systems to enable organisations to demonstrate impact was seen as a key element in the move towards evidencing value. These systems are shaped by an experimental paradigm as their purpose is to generate numerical data to measure performance against prescribed targets (or performance indicators). Generally, the youth workers regarded these new recording systems as intrusive, and felt that they disrupted their 'real' work due to the increasing amount of administration required to fulfil the system requirements as shown in the following quotation:

> *It's becoming harder and harder to be able to do positive work with young people when you're spending so much time justifying why you're doing it.*

For some, the intrusiveness of these systems went deeper, and may be indicative of what Lyotard (1984, cited in Ball 2003) calls the 'terrors of performativity'. In his research on teachers, Ball argued that managerialism created new systems of accountability that were not only about technical and structural reform of organisations but equally focused on reforming teachers and teacher identity. Arguably this can be applied to youth and community workers as demonstrated when one worker said:

> *I think it's a necessary evil now, funding is getting tighter, and funders are getting stricter with what they want. Unfortunately, you have to follow what they say, so it is an absolute pain to get it all done but I think it's going to be one of those things that isn't going to go away.*

The emotive language used by this worker, '*a necessary evil*' and '*an absolute pain*' leave us in no doubt about how he had experienced the new system. Another worker talked about her monthly targets as being '*numbers drilled into my head*'. There is perhaps a degree of resignation that funding comes with 'strings' as one youth worker said:

It's horrible but you're just having to jump through more and more hoops to get the funding so you've got to do what the funding says or else you get nothing at all.

These extracts suggest that the workers saw the monitoring and reporting systems as being for, or belonging to, the funders and managers as opposed to being for, or belonging to, them as practitioners, thus supporting the argument that 'evaluation is in practice predominantly driven by a government performance-driven agenda, and through funding, contractual and regulatory relationships' (Ellis 2009: 7).

Accounting systems are reductionist

Healy (2009) reported on the difficulties faced by the social professions in terms of demonstrating the value of their work through quantitative evaluation processes. Youth workers found the evaluation and recording systems to be reductionist in that they failed to capture the 'real' picture as expressed in the following quotation:

> *They* [monitoring forms] *don't capture half of what you want them to, it's really hard to get that feeling across of someone achieving something that can be really quite small, I remember writing on the form 'attended school for half a day' and thinking if somebody reads that they're going to be like I don't see what the big deal is − but actually for that young person attending school for half a day was huge, they hadn't done it for 6 weeks.*

This extract says something about the sense of frustration arising from the impossibility of trying to capture the complexity of youth and community work on a standardised form. There is concern that the receiver of the information will be unable to comprehend the significance of the youth work intervention from the information provided and hence will be unable to recognise the value of the work. Ball (2003) identifies this as a tension between belief and representation. As Issitt and Spence (2005) argue, monitoring and reporting systems which seek to establish general and universal criteria for measuring 'quality' for purposes of public accountability fail to capture the complexities and subtleties of youth work practice that workers obtain from their interpretation of their experience over time.

Funder-led practice

Funders require evidence of outcomes, of 'value for money' and this is generally sought through a process of prescribed targets. The growth in commissioning and targeted funding has resulted in much youth and community work being about the 'delivery' of packages of learning (Jeffs and Banks 2010). An example of this might be the delivery of issue-based workshops or accreditation aimed at reducing social issues such as anti-social behaviour, obesity or drug and alcohol use. When youth work is constructed as 'packages' of learning, the setting of prescribed outcomes is seen as more plausible; however, this raises some very real concerns about the nature and practice of youth work, particularly in relation to externally imposed targets which direct the focus of practice. One worker talked about the resulting external control of work:

> We have to do work around IAG [Information, Advice and Guidance], drugs and alcohol, sexual health, we have to be doing those because that's what the government wants us to do.

Another worker was clearly uncomfortable with the pressure to 'work on' rather than 'work with' the young person:

> You feel like you have to work with some young people more than others or that you're doing stuff for your own gain to meet those targets rather than working with the young people just because they are the young people that are attending your projects, someone walks in and they say they're NEET [Not in Employment, Education or Training] and you say brilliant, one more tick.

There are indicators here of internal conflicts; 'you feel like you have to work' suggests she feels forced; she is doing this against her will. Her comment, 'You're doing stuff for your own gain', however, suggests that in some way she feels complicit in this action and guilty about working to meet her need to reach targets as opposed to the needs of young people. Another worker spoke about the externally imposed targets directing her work:

> You're pushing young people sometimes in a certain direction to meet the targets of the funding.

Use of the words 'pushing' and 'certain direction' portray a feeling of manipulation of young people which sits awkwardly and uncomfortably with the central values of youth work, in particular participation and empowerment. The requirement to evaluate, record and count 'achievement' can undermine the possibility of developing meaningful relationships with young people (Spence 2004).

These extracts support Spenceley's (2006) assertion that the primary focus of the professional has shifted from the provision of a service to proving the value of the service. The workers' experiences resonate with conclusions drawn by Nias, that the inevitable inability to satisfy one's own conscience and the wider audience leaves professionals 'feeling simultaneously under pressure, guilty and inadequate' (Nias 1989: 193). The final comment 'brilliant, one more tick' has a certain flippancy about it which seemed at odds with the manner of her interview, perhaps a further indicator of her conflicting emotions.

The requirement to accredit young people's engagement in youth work in order to demonstrate its value is a key area of contention. The youth and community workers experienced this as problematic, particularly in relation to how this require-ment was seen to direct their practice. The increased focus on accreditation was often expressed negatively, not so much in terms of accreditation as a concept, but rather accreditation as a focus for youth work. One worker made a link between accreditation and accountability:

> Our targets are things like getting young people through accreditation which is great because it recognises their achievements, but it's because that's the only way we can show funders what we have been doing (...) because there is no way of quantifying the work that you do, so the only way that those funders are going to understand is that that young person then gets a Youth Achievement Award, when actually shoving accreditation down young people's necks is not what they want.

This view that accreditation is used simply because of its ease of measurement reso-nates with a study by Furlong and Cartmel (1997), in which participants also found evaluation mechanisms focused on over-simplistic and easily quantifiable measures. As Spence (2004: 267) states:

> Authenticity implies that youth work cannot be reduced to 'delivering a service'. Services and outcomes are integral but they are only part of the picture. Practice is an interpretative act in which flexibility and openness are crucial.

The following extract illuminates the tension arising from the conflict between the externally imposed output requirement to deliver a number of workshops and these foundational principles of flexibility and openness:

> Part of our targets is to deliver so many workshops on drugs education so we'll do that and a young woman turned round to me the other day and she said 'we just want to chill out' and I was like ... I couldn't say anything to her because we spend all our time saying 'we consult young people, we want to know what you want' and when they say 'we want a space to chill out – we want to be left alone really, we want you to provide activities and give us information if we want it', we go 'that's really cool, that's what you want – NOW we're going to do this!' and I do struggle with that.

There is a real sense of frustration coming through in the way that the worker recounted her experience, particularly when she stated '*I couldn't say anything to her*'. This sense of being rendered speechless may suggest that she did not feel able to respond in a way that she wanted to, in other words she was experiencing a degree of cognitive dissonance, or what Ball (2003) calls 'values schizophrenia' where 'commitment, judgement and authenticity within practice are sacrificed for impres-sion and performance' (ibid.: 221). The worker's discomfort arose from her need to justify her behaviour in terms of the imposition of workshops on young people that opposed her belief in participation and being young people-led.

Tensions between targets and authenticity

Working towards a set of external metrics challenges the ethos of youth and community work, it undermines the quintessential elements of relationship, participation, equity and empowerment. An example of this can be seen in relation to the project's target for establishing new contacts with young people:

> It's about how many young people we engage with and about new young people, I think we just did 140 in the last quarter, and we've got to keep doing that and that's difficult because that's about working with different young people, it's in the back of your mind – I need to move on to new young people to meet those targets.

The phrase '*it's in the back of your mind*' suggests the ongoing tension the worker experienced as a result of trying to meet a target that undermines the relationship aspect of youth work. She is aware that her need to build more and more new relationships will inevitably impact on her existing relationships. The phrase '*I need to move on*' refers implicitly to the need to leave behind those existing relationships as a result of externally imposed targets that appear to take no account of the centrality of relationship in youth work. Starting a relationship with the end in sight has implications for building authentic relationships and this imposed restriction on authenticity may cause youth workers to question their actions in relation to professional values.

This concern was shared by another worker; this worker was more explicit in identifying the possible impact of a contact numbers target on existing relationships:

> I've got quite high contact numbers and I'm going to spend my time moving provision around to ensure that I hit that number of young people but what about the young people that we've already engaged with? What – we've got their details we can now push them to the side – we don't.

The interesting point here is expressed in the final phrase '*we don't*' as this indicates an agentic response to managing the target culture. Evans (2008) argues that professionals do not passively accept externally imposed changes to practice; rather they are potentially key players in shaping their professional practice. Furbey, Reid and Cole (2001) also argue that individuals can adapt, adopt, resist or circumnavigate external demands for change. There was limited talk about how the youth workers did this. Only two other workers in the study mentioned how:

> I don't let them [targets] stop me doing the work I want to do, I do the work I want to do, that young people want us to do and then just make it fit the targets afterwards. You manage it in the best way you can, you learn ways to sort of, I guess, manipulate the targets.

These extracts suggest that these youth workers had adopted a 'strategic compliance' position (Gleeson and Shain 1999) towards the changes imposed upon them by the external funding requirements. In other words, these workers demonstrated a recognition and acceptance of the non-negotiable aspects, but had developed ways to work around these that enable them to maintain their professional values and commitment to the young people.

This raises questions about why there is not more evidence of workers' achieving agency, of manipulating 'the system' in favour of meeting young people's needs rather than external funders' requirements (Emirbayer and Mische 1998). It may be that the factors that enable professionals to act with agency have been eroded or undermined. However, this link was not explicitly made by the youth and community workers themselves. Osgood (2006) argues that practitioners need sufficient belief in themselves as professionals to challenge top-down change and perhaps, as with the early-years workers in her study, some of the workers in this study felt powerless to resist.

Tensions between targets and values

Arguably, the ability of workers to adhere to youth and community work principles is being eroded by the growth of the contract culture. One worker raised the question of how far youth work can go in terms of meeting funder requirements before it compromises itself to such an extent it can no longer be called youth work, he asked:

> *Are things getting overlooked because we're actually having to concentrate on what the funders want rather than what young people want and need? They've given us all of this money but what do we have to do for it, and that is the thing that I am hating at the moment about the way things are going and it's only going to get worse.*

Another worker identified the challenge at a more personal level:

> *I think we get pushed out of our comfort zones and why we went into the job in the first place, yes, we bring in funding which is important, but at the expense of what really?*

She highlights the question for her in relation to her 'calling' to youth work, in other words her professional *raison d'être*. This resonates strongly with Nias's (1989) findings in relation to the challenges professionals face in terms of balancing competing demands and conflicting values. Mahony and Hextall's (2000) concern that professional autonomy and morale were being eroded by the privileging of accountability-focused evaluation processes appears to be valid. The sense of challenge or threat to professional values supports Reinders's (2008) assertion that managerialism has brought about the 'invasion of a different set of values' into professional practices. The youth workers were indeed seriously struggling to remain faithful to their professional values. The experience of these youth workers also resonates with those in the study by Edward, Coffield, Steer and Gregson (2007) in the sense that they find themselves trying to meet conflicting demands while also trying to reconcile these demands with their own professional values, as well as with their own priorities for the work that they do. Challenge to one's values goes to the very core of 'identity', of who people are and how they feel about themselves and what they do; this is significant in terms of achieving agency. There are similarities between the data here and Spenceley's (2006) study of professionalism in the Further Education (FE) sector, particularly with regard to practitioners feeling they are no longer in control of the design of their work, and rather that this had been taken from them by external forces, namely the economy. She used the term 'servant of the economy' to describe the re-positioning of FE and the imposition of various government agendas; my analysis suggests this could be equally applied to youth work.

The question of whose needs should be prioritised, the funders or a young person is clearly a tension for the youth workers in this study, reflecting Bernstein's (1996) assertion that performativity results in 'contract replacing covenant'. Ball (2003: 226) uses the phrase 'process of exteriorisation' to describe the shift in the relationship between the practitioner and her/his work, arguing that a commitment to 'service' no longer has value or meaning and professional judgement is subordinated to the requirements of performativity and marketing. This tension can be seen in the articulation of self-questioning by the youth and community workers as to where their work seemed to be heading. They ask, for example: What are we doing? Are we doing what we were doing before? Is it what we came into the profession to do? Do we believe in what we are doing? Again, this attunes with Ball's study, particularly the question he raised: 'Do we value who we are able to be, who we are becoming in the labyrinth of performativity?' (Ball 2003: 220).

The ways in which the youth workers managed the tensions was interesting as it raised questions as to their level of compliance. Drawing on Gleeson and Shain's (1999) typology of compliance – willing, unwilling and strategic – it would seem that the majority of the youth workers adopted 'strategic' compliance: 'a form of artful pragmatism which reconciles professional and managerial interests' (Gleeson and Shain 1999: 482). Workers have to balance the requirements of funders with their own values, and seek as far as possible to work with the needs and agendas of the young people (Tyler 2009). Many youth and community workers are attempting to successfully negotiate these competing priorities, as shown by the extracts in this chapter and within other studies (see Spence, Devanney and Noonan 2006; and Davies and Merton 2009). On the whole they found ways to retain their professional values while accepting the fact that some aspects of the new work culture were non-negotiable. They sought ways to work around these conditions in the interests of the young people. This position requires continued internal and external negotiation and will be accompanied by a sense of continual flux, instability and uncertainty, all of which demand effort and energy and can be emotionally draining.

In summary, this chapter has drawn on empirical research to present the argument that practitioners can feel alienated from the process of evaluation because it appears incompatible with the nature of their work. The youth workers expressed frustration in relation to the fact that they had no control over what constituted a successful outcome. The removal of the opportunity to make and record professional judgements by the introduction of standardised tick-box forms undermined their sense of professionalism. The quasi-experimental evaluation system was flawed in terms of enabling the practitioners to fully and accurately account for their work. An even more serious concern is that it had the potential to distort the work as the requirements of the funders became paramount. The purpose of youth work, in regards to challenging inequalities and injustices and addressing the concerns of people and groups whose voices are unheard, is severely undermined in this context. In these austere times, when resources are scarce, there is arguably a need for a sharper focus on the demonstration of 'value for money', however, the inadequacy of an accountability-focused process to demonstrate this 'value' is clear.

References

Ball, S. (2003) 'The Teacher's Soul and the Terrors of Performativity', in *Journal of Education Policy*, Vol. 18(2), pp. 215–228

Bernstein, B. (1996) *Pedagogy Symbolic Control and Identity*, London: Taylor & Francis

Brent, G. (2004) 'The Arch and the Smile', in *Youth & Policy*, Vol. 84, pp 69–73

Cooper, S. (2012) 'Transformative Evaluation: An Interpretive Study of Youth Workers' Experience of Using Participatory Evaluation', Doctoral Thesis, available at https://ore.exeter.ac.uk/repository/handle/10036/3759

Davies, B. and Merton, B. (2009) 'Squaring the Circle? Findings of a 'Modest Inquiry' into the State of Youth Work Practice in a Changing Policy Environment' accessed at www.dmu.ac.uk/documents/health-and-life-sciences-documents/research/squaringthecircle.pdf (24.02.17)

Edward, S., Coffield, F., Steer, R. and Gregson, M. (2007) 'Endless Change in the Learning and Skills Sector: The Impact on Teaching Staff', in *Journal of Vocational Education & Training*, Vol. 59(2), pp.155–173

Ellis, J. (2009) 'Monitoring and Evaluation in the Third Sector: Meeting Accountability and Learning Needs', paper delivered at the 15th NCVO/VSSN Researching the Voluntary Sector Conference 2009

Emirbayer, M. and Mische, A. (1998) 'What Is Agency?', in *American Journal of Sociology*, Vol. 103(4), pp. 962–1023

Evans, L. (2008) 'Professionalism, Professionality and the Development of Education Professionals', in *British Journal of Educational Studies*, Vol. 56(1), pp. 20–38

Everitt, A. and Hardiker, P. (1996) *Evaluating for Good Practice*, Basingstoke: Palgrave

Furbey, R., Reid, B. and Cole, I. (2001) 'Housing Professionalism in the United Kingdom: The Final Curtain or a New Age?' in *Housing, Theory and Society*, Vol. 18, pp. 36–49

Furlong, A. and Cartmel, F. (1997) *Evaluating Youth Work with Vulnerable Young People, SCRE Research Report No. 83,* The Scottish Council for Research in Education

Gleeson, D. and Shain, F. (1999) 'Managing Ambiguity: Between Markets and Managerialism – A Case Study of "Middle" Managers in Further Education', in *The Sociological Review*, Vol. 47(3), pp. 461–490

Healy, K. (2009) 'A Case of Mistaken Identity: The Social Welfare Professions and New Public Management', in *Journal of Sociology*, Vol. 45, pp. 401–418

Issitt, M. and Spence, J. (2005) 'Practitioner Knowledge and Evidence-based Research, Policy and Practice', in *Youth & Policy* Vol. 88, pp. 63–82

Jeffs, T. and Banks, S. (2010) 'Youth Workers as Controllers: Issues of Method and Purpose', in S. Banks (ed.) *Ethical Issues in Youth Work*, London: Routledge, pp. 106–122

Mahony, P. and Hextall, I. (2000) *Reconstructing Teaching*, London: Routledge Falmer

Nias, J. (1989) *Primary Teachers Talking: A Study of Teaching as Work*, London: Routledge

Ord, J. (2007) *Youth Work Process, Product and Practice: Creating an Authentic Curriculum in Work with Young People*, Lyme Regis: RHP

Osgood, J. (2006) 'Professionalism and Performativity: The Feminist Challenge Facing Early Years Practitioners', in *Early Years*, Vol. 26(2), pp. 187–199

Reinders, H. (2008) 'The Transformation of Human Services', in *Journal of Intellectual Disability Research*, Vol. 52(7), pp. 564–572

Spence, J. (2004) 'Targeting, Accountability and Youth Work Practice', in *Practice*, Vol. 16(4), pp. 261–272

Spence, J., Devanney, C. and Noonan, K. (2006) *Youth Work: Voices of Practice*, Leicester: National Youth Agency

Spenceley, L. (2006) '"Smoke and Mirrors": An Examination of the Concept of Professionalism within the FE Sector', in *Research in Post-Compulsory Education*, Vol. 11(3), pp. 289–302

Tyler, M. (2009) 'Managing the Tensions', in J. Wood and J. Hine (eds), *Work With Young People*, London: Sage Publications, pp. 233–246

Watson, D. and Emery, C. (2010) 'From Rhetoric to Reality: The Problematic Nature and Assessment of Children and Young People's Social and Emotional Learning', in *British Educational Research Journal*, Vol. 36(5), pp. 767–786

PART 2
Participatory evaluation

Participatory evaluation is an approach that offers many advantages to those involved in youth and community work. These include enhanced access to information, deep and rich data and the opportunity to develop shared understandings. There is close alignment between participatory evaluation and youth and community work ethos, values and practice. This supports the engagement of practitioners, young people and communities in the process of evaluation. Importantly, participatory evaluation approaches can also support a clear articulation of what youth and community work is and demonstrate what it can achieve to a wider audience.

The opening chapter in this part of the book ('What is participatory evaluation?') introduces the reader to the concept of participatory evaluation and presents an overview of the histories, rationale, purpose and underpinning principles. Focus is given to the critical exploration of the central issues of participation and power. The chapter concludes by making a case for using participatory approaches in the evaluation of youth work, highlighting the congruence between values and practice principles.

Chapter 5 ('Participatory evaluation approaches') explores in detail a range of approaches; namely empowerment evaluation, collaborative evaluation and democratic evaluation. All these approaches centralise stakeholder involvement; yet there are differences between them and the current debates around these are discussed. Practice models are presented for each approach to further illustrate how these approaches address issues of involvement and participation.

Chapter 6 ('Transformative Evaluation') presents a participatory approach developed by the author specifically for the youth and community work context. This approach is currently being used in a range of contexts and settings in England, Scotland, France, Italy, Estonia, Finland and Australia. The rationale and theoretical foundations of this approach are explained in detail. The four stage model is described and its associated advantages and disadvantages are discussed.

The concluding chapter ('Learning in participatory evaluation') focuses on the potentiality of the participatory paradigm in relation to the learning and knowledge generation function of evaluation. The argument is made that participatory evaluation can be a tool for learning as well as a tool for judging value. The various ways in which participatory evaluation provides learning opportunities for practitioners, participants, organisations and ultimately policy-makers and funders are presented. This chapter concludes with a proposition that participatory evaluation supports practitioner involvement, and through this, they develop their confidence and agency. Ultimately, participatory evaluation approaches offer those involved in youth and community work a more appropriate means of identifying and communicating the value of their work.

4

WHAT IS PARTICIPATORY EVALUATION?

Introduction

Participatory evaluation is perhaps best understood as an approach to evaluation rather than a specific method. In essence, it is a process of collective action that involves a range of stakeholders in reflection, negotiation, collaboration and knowledge creation. There are a number of types of evaluation that come under the umbrella of participatory evaluation and these differ in terms of the form of participation and the choice of stakeholders. In other words, they differ in relation to whose participation is sought and how participation is understood. This chapter begins by discussing the defining characteristics of participatory evaluation. This leads into an exploration of its underpinning philosophy and values and evolutionary developments. The related concepts of participation and empowerment, fundamental to participatory evaluation, are examined in depth. The chapter concludes by making the case for participatory evaluation in the context of youth and community work.

Defining participatory evaluation

It is important to state from the outset that participatory evaluation is not simply a matter of using participatory techniques, it is about rethinking who initiates and undertakes the process and who learns or benefits from the findings (Guijt and Gaventa 1998). A focus on process is one of the defining characteristics of participatory evaluation (Whitmore 1991), and Jackson and Kassam (1998) describe this process as one that:

- empowers individuals, communities and organisations to analyse and solve their own problems;
- values the knowledge and experience of participants;

- uses learning to promote reflection and critical analysis by project participants and practitioners;
- seeks to improve the programme and the organisation in the interests of the users;
- uses participatory methods of obtaining data and generating knowledge, employing a diversity of methods (predominantly qualitative but sometimes quantitative); and
- is participatory and collective and aims to create a more in-depth and accurate knowledge of the performance and impacts of practice interventions.

Clearly, learning is at the centre of this process. Suárez-Herrera, Springett and Kagan (2009: 323) assert that 'those who learn from evaluation are those who do evaluation'. It is important, therefore, to interrogate any approach claiming to be participatory by asking the key question of who benefits from the learning and how?

Through engaging in participatory evaluation, stakeholders learn more about the organisation and about themselves in the context and situation in which they are participating. Context is an important aspect and as Cousins, Whitmore and Shulha (2012) point out, it is often overlooked by a desire for rigour in conventional evaluation approaches and designs. They argue that failing to take account of context can diminish the learning function of evaluation and restrict the role of evaluation in programme development. If learning and change are to become the focus of the evaluation process, extended involvement and collaboration between stakeholders is required, as is openness to dialogue, critical reflection and negotiation.

There are clear differences between participatory evaluation and experimental evaluation. They have different purposes. The purpose of participatory evaluation is not only concerned with tracking change in those directly involved in the intervention but also about ensuring that learning travels up organisational hierarchies and brings about change there as well. The advantages of using a participatory approach are that it sets out to acknowledge and elevate the perspectives, voices, and decisions of the least powerful and the most affected stakeholders (Jackson and Kassam 1998). It promotes a 'doing with' rather than a 'doing to' paradigm and it recognises the importance of people's participation in analysing and interpreting change, that is, learning from experience.

While it is often the case that participatory evaluation generates qualitative data, it is a misconception that it only uses this; it can also include quantitative approaches to data generation (Guijt 2014). There has been a growth in participatory approaches that generate quantitative data (Chambers 2007). If quantitative data is to be used to inform participatory evaluation, it is important to ensure the participation of relevant stakeholders in some or all of the following actions: the design of data collection tools, the generation of data and the analysis of the data (see Part 3 for further discussion).

Underpinning philosophy and values

Chambers (1995) identified the shift in philosophy, a move from a paradigm of things to a paradigm of people, as a trigger for the evolution of participatory evaluation. Guba and Lincoln (1989: 183) argue that the positivist paradigm of evaluation is 'linear and closed' and promote participatory evaluation for its ability to be 'iterative, interactive, hermeneutic, at times intuitive and almost certainly open'. Participatory evaluation sits within the interpretive paradigm (see Chapter 1) as it recognises that knowledge is a social construction, that people construct their 'lived' reality by attaching specific meanings to their experience, and that this construction will result in multiple versions of 'reality' (Denzin and Lincoln 2005).

Participatory evaluation takes account of the importance of context in shaping people's realities. It aims to explore these multiple perspectives in an attempt to develop shared meanings. It supports a more democratic and political approach to evaluation in that it raises questions about who defines and measures change and for whose benefit this is done (Estrella 2000). The very fact that it is participatory implies democracy (Ledwith and Springett 2010), that people have a voice in the decisions that affect their lives and act collectively for the common good. Greene (in Ryan 1998: 109) states that participatory evaluation is underpinned by a value commitment to democratic pluralism that aims 'to broadening the policy conversation to include all legitimate perspectives and voices, and to full and fair stakeholder participation in policy and program decision-making.' An analysis of power is required to enable this commitment to democracy. This analysis needs to be informed by a commitment to social justice and the pursuit of social change with, and on behalf of, vulnerable and oppressed individuals and groups within society. Participatory evaluation presupposes that knowledge is a potential source of power, and as such, it should not be exclusively owned by those in power.

In summary, participatory evaluation is a value-based practice that seeks to serve the needs of a range of stakeholders, including participants, practitioners and organisations and funders. It explicitly raises questions in relation to the political economy of evaluation such as 'Who would gain? Who might lose? And how? And, especially, how was it intended and anticipated that the findings would make a difference' (Chambers 2009: 4). Where there is a commitment to participatory practice, evaluation can significantly contribute to empowerment by centralising the voice of all involved, although this is not guaranteed. It cannot be assumed that just because something is called 'participatory', it is empowering. In order to meet the empowerment aim it is necessary to critically consider how meaningful participation of a range of stakeholders can be achieved.

Developments in participatory evaluation

The concept of participatory evaluation emerged in the 1930s. Its origin is in the field of development studies, with much of the early literature coming from Latin

America, Africa and Asia. It developed from participatory research (PR) which, according to Maguire (1987), was a response to two critiques of international economic development work at that time: a growing appreciation of adult education as empowerment and the increasing challenge to the dominant experimental paradigm to adequately account for the work. In essence, participatory research involves a combination of three activities: investigation, education and action (known as Participatory Action Research). Participatory research has an explicit political aim in that it seeks to:

- promote change through the raising of critical consciousness in the researcher and participants;
- bring about improvements in the lives of those involved; and
- transform basic social structures and relationships.

A more holistic, pluralist and egalitarian worldview was emerging in which people were seen as 'co-creating their reality through participation: through their experience, their imagination and intuition, their thinking and their action' (Reason 1994: 324). This worldview supported a different set of assumptions and paved the way for participatory research (and evaluation). These predispositions took account of the political nature of research and evaluation and challenged the dominant view that inquiry could be neutral or context-free. Questions were raised about who can create valid knowledge and the notion of 'expert' was critiqued. In response, a view that ordinary people are capable of generating knowledge that is as important and as valid as that produced by scientific processes gained ground.

In the late 1960s and 1970s development agencies began to associate failure of development efforts with the lack of consideration of local realities, including social, cultural, political and environmental factors that affected both the feasibility and sustainability of programmes. A new approach to development that took account of and valued local knowledge and experience in shaping project design was deemed necessary. Chambers (1995), often seen as an originator of participatory evaluation, developed a process called Rapid Rural Appraisal (RRA) which sought to involve participants in gathering data to inform project designs. This process evolved further as participants were given authority for generating data themselves, and thus Participatory Rural Appraisal (PRA) took hold. While Chambers's work was driven by practical needs, it was ideology that was the driving force behind the work of Fals-Borda. Drawing on the work of Freire (1970), *Pedagogy of the Oppressed*, he advocated for participatory evaluation because he viewed it as a political act capable of calling disadvantaged people to take actions against exploitation (Fals-Borda and Rahman 1991).

A number of participatory evaluation approaches have developed in response to a growing need for evaluations to be more inclusive, more culturally responsive and to take account of the complex needs of communities, programmes and programme interventions. Chouinard and Milley (2016) identified over forty different methods and argued that while these have much in common, they can generally be differentiated in terms of rationale, ideological predispositions and the depth and nature of stakeholder involvement. The Cousins and Whitmore (1998) framework provides a helpful guide when trying to differentiate the different approaches. This framework classifies approaches as either Practical Participatory Evaluation (PPE) or as Transformative Participatory Evaluation (TPE). Practical participatory evaluation is predominantly concerned with programme problem solving and increasing the use of evaluation for decision-making whereas transformative participatory evaluation is driven by emancipatory and political purposes and has its focus on social change.

The Cousins and Whitmore model has been critiqued, particularly in relation to how stakeholder involvement is envisaged and enabled, and further refinements have been made. For example, Toal (2009) specified a range of different stakeholder activities in the process and Cullen, Coryn and Rugh (2011) introduce the concept of phases within the evaluation process, rather than particular tasks or activities, to take account of the temporal nature of stakeholder participation. Rather than seeing the two streams (PPE and TPE) as a framework into which all participatory evaluation approaches can be situated, it may be that this useful distinction can be applied beneficially to each approach. For example, Fetterman and Wandersman (2007) argued that empowerment evaluation can be practical, transformative or both depending on the purpose for which it is being used. Chapter 5 explores three participatory approaches – empowerment evaluation, collaborative evaluation and democratic evaluation – in more detail. The relational and dialogical nature of participatory evaluation represents a significant difference to the experimental approach and while there is clearly variation between the many participatory approaches, they are united by two central features: participation and a value commitment to democratic pluralism. They aim to include all legitimate perspectives and voices in the evaluation process.

Participation and empowerment

Participation and empowerment emerged as popular terms in social policy towards the end of the twentieth century, reflecting the focus in western society at that time on social inclusion, citizen rights and responsibilities and participatory democracy. Participation can be understood from two standpoints. Taking a participatory democracy worldview standpoint, participation can be viewed as giving voice to the most marginalised and supporting communities to be in control of the decision-making processes that affect their lives. In this context, participation can be seen as transformative, for example, Ledwith and Springett (2010: 13) describe participation as 'a way of life, a way of seeing the world and a way of being in the world'. This interpretation is underpinned by commitments to justice and equity and a belief in the worth of everyone. From a radical standpoint, participation can be understood as a struggle against political and economic exclusion, focusing on exercising control over and access to public resources (Fals–Borda 1998). This interpretation is underpinned by the idea that communities should be empowered to exert direct influence in decisions that impact on their social, material and environmental well-being. Participation is widely believed to be a good thing, a basic need and a democratic right.

In the context of young people, the United Nations *Convention on the Rights of the Child* (1989) brought a shift in the way children were viewed and treated, from being passive 'objects' of care to human beings with a distinct set of rights. Article 12 states that every child has the right to say what they think in all matters affecting them, and to have their views taken seriously. Groundwater-Smith, Dockett and Bottrell (2015) argue that while actions have been taken internationally to create mechanisms for young people's views to be heard, for example, the appointment of Children's Commissioners in England, there is less evidence that change has occurred in areas such as education, health and youth justice. One reason for this may be that there is still much confusion about what 'participation' and 'empowerment' mean.

White, Sadanandan Nair and Ashcroft (1994) used the analogy of participation as a kaleidoscope, suggesting that participation changes depending on who controls it; it is fragile, illusive and ever-changing. In essence it is argued that these terms (participation and empowerment) can mean different things to different people, at different times. However, it is risky to uncritically accept participation and empowerment as a good thing as this can mask their political nature (Beresford 2005). Cooke and Kothari (2001) questioned the common assumption that participation is automatically 'a good thing' arguing that it is all too often treated as if it is a technical matter. If the political nature of participation is ignored, it can become a tool to serve the needs of those in power.

Participation and consultation are often seen as related but Hill, Davis, Prout and Tisdall (2004: 83) assert that they should not be seen as synonymous, arguing that while 'consultation may be a means of enabling children to participate ... it can also be a substitute for participation in that decisions are made without the direct involvement of children'. Lansdown (2005) makes a distinction based on the different levels of young people's engagement in relation to participatory research, this can be applied to participatory evaluation as shown in Table 4.1.

In the context of youth and community work, Ord (2007) states that participation can be understood as a combination of four interrelated factors. He identifies these as responsibility, decision-making, engagement and action. He argues that in order to participate, young people need to take responsibility for their involvement and, as far as possible, be involved in relevant decision-making in relation to the object of participation. These two factors (responsibility and decision-making) determine the level of the third factor – engagement, and ultimately their participation must result in some action. Fitzsimons, Hope, Russell and Cooper (2011) suggest that empowerment can be understood as a strategy and as a process; a strategy for including people in decision-making processes and an internal process whereby individual young people develop and through this development, change their self concept.

TABLE 4.1 Levels of engagement

Consultation	Recognition that young people's perspectives make a valuable contribution.	Seeks to elicit information from young people to be used by adults.	Process is driven by adults.
Participatory process	Seeks to develop partnerships between young people and adults.	Young people are involved in development, implementation, monitoring and evaluation phases of the project.	Young people have the opportunity to shape the agenda.
Self-initiated process	Young people adopt the role of evaluator (facilitated by adults).	Young people are empowered to take action, they define the agenda and actions to be taken.	Process is driven by young people.

Ord and Fitzsimons et al. both agree that participation and empowerment are interconnected, that one relies on the other – a young person may not be able to participate in an empowering strategy unless they perceive themselves able to do so. This links with the notion of agency, which can be understood as 'the ability of individuals or groups to act on their situations, to behave as subjects rather than objects in their own lives, to shape their own circumstances and ultimately achieve change' (Jeffrey 2011:6).

The nature of power is slippery and ambiguous (Mullender, Ward and Fleming 2013). Early conceptions of power as an entity that could be possessed, as something you either have or do not have, have been challenged. This has allowed us to move beyond 'zero-sum' thinking in relation to power, where a gain for one person entails a corresponding loss for the other.

According to Foucault (1975) power is better conceived of as relational, it exists in the relationships between people. For Giddens (1984) power resides in individuals. Both viewed power itself as neutral. Giddens believes that power, within the dialectical relationship between people and society, has the capacity to transform the structure of society. When power is conceived as a process as well as an outcome, as interactive rather than as an oppressive force, we can see that empowerment is something that we claim for ourselves rather than something that is done to us. Two enabling factors need to be present; firstly, we need to believe in the possibility of change and secondly, we need to believe that we possess the power to bring that change about. If we are to promote and enable participation we need to recognise that young people are capable of making choices, and are worthy of respect (Jeffrey 2011).

Young people's participation can be interpreted in different ways. Importantly, the level to which they are able to participate depends on *both* their ability and capacity to participate, *and* the way in which the adults working with them interpret the term 'participation'. Arguably, there are few genuine opportunities for young people to participate in self-initiated processes and much participation occurs at the level of system-maintaining rather than the system-transforming (Lansdown 2005). Inherent difficulties exist in contexts that simultaneously seek to liberate and constrain young people and their behaviour (Christensen and James [2008] cited in Groundwater-Smith et al. 2015: 11). Despite good intentions, the practice of participation often falls short of its ideals and expectations. Meaningful participation requires the participant to experience and to be viewed as the subject rather than the object of understanding (Froggett 2002). It is not sufficient to simply advocate participation, as Graham and Harris (2005: 106) argue, we must be participatory:

> Being participatory involves more than using a particular technique or approach. It reflects an attitude towards human interaction. It means exhibiting a willingness to share decision-making and power.

Beresford (2005) identified a number of concerns coming from service-users and service-user organisations, particularly in relation to the ideological basis of participation. He identifies two approaches to participation (see Table 4.2), and argues that because the differences between these two approaches have not been made explicit, the consumerist approach to participation has been allowed to dominate in public policy.

Models of participation

There are a number of models of participation, but perhaps the most well-known are Arnstein's 'Ladder of Citizen Participation' (1969) and Hart's Ladder (1992). The first was developed for use in community settings and the second for young

TABLE 4.2 Consumerist and democratic approaches to participation (from Beresford 2005)

Approach	Consumerist	Democratic
Drivers	The introduction of market-driven approaches to public services (managerialism).	A concern with people having greater control over their lives and the services that affect them.
Emphasis	Service-user as customer.	Focus on inclusion, autonomy and independence.
Power dimension	Apolitical – does not seek to redistribute power or locus of decision-making.	Explicitly political – highlights issues of power and is committed to redistribution of power.
Conception of participation	Participation is an information-gathering tool for those in power to shape policy and provision.	Participation is a liberatory process, committed to personal and political change and empowerment.

people's participation. Both models differentiate eight levels of participation. The two bottom rungs in Arnstein's model are:

1.   manipulation
2.   therapy

These are described as non-participation as it is argued that the purpose of these levels is not to enable people to participate in planning or delivery of programmes, but to support organisations to provide a service. The next three rungs are:

3.   informing
4.   consultation
5.   placation

These levels are described as tokenism as while they allow service-users to have a voice and to advise, they do not promote any real power-sharing. The top three rungs are:

6.   partnership
7.   delegated power
8.   citizen control

These levels represent participation that involves increasing degrees of power sharing.

Hart's Ladder also has eight rungs; he terms the first three rungs manipulation, decoration and tokenism as all describe levels of non-participation. Five further rungs (assigned but informed, consulted and informed, adult-initiated – shared decisions with youth, youth-initiated – shared decisions with adults, and youth-initiated and directed) describe ascending levels of participation.

Both models have proved to be useful in practice, but equally, they have been critiqued on the basis that they are linear and hierarchical and thus fail to recognise the complex and dynamic nature of participation. The use of a ladder implicitly suggests that getting to the top is the ultimate aim, but the desired level of participation surely depends on the nature and purpose of the activity. In reality, one level may not necessarily lead to the next and both models are context-free. In an attempt to address the shortcomings of a linear model and the complex and contextual nature of participation, Treseder (1997) adapted Hart's Ladder, to present the five forms of participation (assigned but informed, consulted and informed, adult-initiated – shared decisions with youth, youth-initiated – shared decisions with adults, and youth-initiated and directed) as a circular model. These, he argued, should be regarded as five different, but equal forms of good practice and that the 'best' approach was whatever was the most appropriate for the context and situation. Table 4.3 summarises how these forms of participation can be understood in relation to participatory evaluation.

TABLE 4.3 Forms of young people's participation in participatory evaluation

Assigned but informed	The evaluation is designed and implemented by adults. Young people volunteer to be involved and to share their experience/ understanding with the evaluator. They understand the nature of their involvement (who decided to involve them and why). Their input is valued and their views are respected.
Consulted and informed	The evaluation is designed and run by adults, but young people are consulted about the aspects they are involved in. They have a full understanding of the evaluation processes to be used and their opinions about these are taken on board.
Adult-initiated, shared decisions with young people	The evaluation is designed by adults who set the parameters. Young people are involved in decision-making in relation to the planning and implementation of the evaluation.
Young people-initiated, shared decisions with adults	Young people are involved in the design stage of the evaluation. They work collaboratively with adults to make decisions about how the evaluation will be implemented. The adults act as mentors, offering expertise and support.
Young people-initiated and directed	Young people are involved in the design stage of the evaluation. They decide on how the evaluation is to be carried out. Adults are available to support, provide training and resources.

Making the case for participatory evaluation in youth and community work

There are four typical arguments to support participation in evaluation (Gregory 2000). Firstly, an argument based on ethics, that it is the 'right' thing to do. This is premised on a belief that being involved in decision-making in relation to things that affect us is a human right. Secondly, that it is expedient, it makes sense at a practical level in that if people are not involved in decision-making they may revoke or subvert decisions made by others. A third argument is that participation enables effective decision-making as it involves all those considered to be 'experts' in the service or provision being evaluated. The expert knowledge (lived experience) of service-users is valuable. The fourth argument is that participation in decision-making means that people are aware of and understand the rationale for any decision made and are thus more likely to support its implementation. As Sillitoe (2002 :5) argues, participatory evaluation can provide 'ways to facilitate others' expression of their understanding of the rapidly changing world while informing them of our thoughts'. This can lead to mutual comprehension. The argument for using participatory evaluation approaches in youth and community work is further supported by one of alignment. It follows that because youth and community work is committed to education, empowerment and participation, then the approach to evaluating it should mirror this. If the evaluation approach fits the organisation's philosophy, this should enhance the likelihood of it being accepted, carried out and bearing impact.

TABLE 4.4 Benefits of using participatory evaluation (adapted from Mullinix and Akalsa-Bukachi 1998: 168)

Area	Participants gains	Organisation gains
Origin of purpose	The interests and priorities of the participants shape the evaluation questions.	Greater understanding of the needs of the community. Helps to ensure that aims and objectives are set according to need. Increases likelihood of achieving success.
Extended usefulness	An understanding of the purpose and importance of evaluation and the ability to conduct meaningful evaluations.	Increased likelihood of collecting relevant and appropriate information. Increases ability to be accountable.
Skills development	Develop the ability to collect, analyse and act on information.	Cost-effective. Sustainability.
Locus of control	Participants empowered to take responsibility for assessing and articulating the impact a project has had on them according to their priorities.	Sustainability. Increases ability to be accountable.

The benefits of participatory evaluation are multidimensional. Mullinix and Akalsa-Bukachi (1998), drawing on their work with Kenyan women, identify four distinctive areas in which the participants benefit; this can be further extended to show the benefit for youth and community work organisations as shown in Table 4.4.

Engaging in participatory evaluation enables practitioners to examine the politics, values, and normative aspect of their practice. It promotes an attitude and outlook that encourages workers to listen to other people's stories, to be attentive to alternative view points, and to be aware of and considerate to new ways of seeing and doing. This outlook supports workers to continually challenge their own generalised assumptions and those of their peers. If we see this as an essential aspect of the youth and community worker's role, then the affinity between the participatory evaluation and youth and community work is obvious. As shown in Table 4.4, young people also benefit from being involved in participatory evaluation. This in itself is beneficial for workers as young people are more able to recognise and articulate their learning and their engagement further develops existing relationships between young people and youth workers (see Chapter 7 for a more detailed discussion).

Summary

Over the past thirty years or so, youth and community workers have been put under great pressure to provide evidence of outcomes in an attempt to prove the changes their work makes to the lives of young people and communities. Many have argued that the dominance of the experimental paradigm has compromised their work (Smith 2001; Issitt and Spence 2005; Cooper 2011). Participatory forms of evaluation can provide a form of resistance to the dominant discourse of evaluation as a technology of power (Everitt and Hardiker 1996). Adopting participatory evaluation approaches offers practitioners and organisations an opportunity to reclaim the evaluation agenda as a process for improving practice. It can provide an antidote to the 'the negative side-effects of target-driven action – both in programme performance and evaluation practice' (Elliott and Kushner 2007: 326).

However, the question of whether participatory evaluation can respond to the needs of accountability-based management must be raised. Early promoters made the case that it could (Jackson and Kassam 1998; Estrella 2000), yet the impact of participatory evaluation is rarely seen at the macro level and there is little evidence of its effects on policy-making (Kemshall and Littlechild 2000). This, however, should not deter us. There is a growing interest within the context of youth and community work, and the positive effects of participatory evaluation at the micro level (in the activity between service-user and front-line worker), and at mezo level (in relation to organisational decision-making) are evident. These positive effects create enthusiasm and energy and have the potential to encourage others to adopt participatory approaches, creating a snowball effect. An increase in the use of participatory approaches will support the development of a robust evidence-base that ultimately will impact at the policy level.

References

Arnstein, S. (1969) 'A Ladder of Citizen Participation', in *Journal of the American Institute of Planners*, 35, pp. 216–224, accessed at http://lithgow-schmidt.dk/sherry-arnstein/ladder-of-citizen-participation.html (10.03.16)

Beresford, P. (2005) 'Service-user Involvement in Evaluation and Research: Issues, Dilemmas and Destinations', in D. Taylor and S. Balloch (eds), *The Politics of Evaluation*, Bristol: The Policy Press, pp. 77–85

Chambers, R. (2009) 'So that the Poor Count More: Using Participatory Methods for Impact Evaluation', in R. Chambers, D. Karlan, M. Ravallion and P. Rogers, *Designing Impact Evaluations: Different Perspectives, Working Paper 4*, New Delhi: International Initiative for Impact Evaluation, accessed at http://betterevaluation.org/resource/over view/Designing_impact_evaluations_different_perspectives (15.03.16)

Chambers, R. (2007) *Who Counts? The Quiet Revolution of Participation and Numbers*, Working Paper 296, Brighton: The Institute of Development Studies, accessed at www. ids.ac.uk/files/Wp296.pdf (10.03.16)

Chambers, R. (1995) 'Paradigm Shifts and the Practice of Participatory Research and Development', in N. Nelson and S. Wright (eds), *Power and Participatory Development: Theory and Practice*, London: Intermediate Technology Publications, pp. 30–42

Chouinard, J. and Milley, P. (2016) 'Mapping the Spatial Dimensions of Participatory Practice: A Discussion of Context in Evaluation', in *Evaluation and Program Planning*, 54, pp. 1–10

Cooke, B. and Kothari, U. (eds) (2001) *Participation: The New Tyranny*, London: Zed Books

Cooper, S. (2011) 'Reconnecting with Evaluation: The Benefits of Using a Participatory Approach to Assess Impact', in *Youth & Policy*, Vol. 107, pp. 55–70

Cousins, J.B. and Whitmore, E. (1998) 'Framing Participatory Evaluation', in E. Whitmore (ed.), *Understanding and Practicing Participatory Evaluation*, San Francisco: Jossey-Bass, pp. 5–23

Cousins, J.B., Whitmore, E. and Shulha, L. (2012) 'Arguments for a Common Set of Principles for Collaborative Inquiry in Evaluation', *American Journal of Evaluation*, Vol. 34(1), pp. 7–22

Cullen, A., Coryn, C. and Rugh, J. (2011) 'The politics and consequences of including stakeholders in international development evaluation', in *American Journal of Evaluation*, Vol. 32(3), pp. 345–361

Denzin, N. and Lincoln, Y. (eds) (2005) *The Sage Handbook of Qualitative Research* (3rd ed.), London: Sage Publications

Elliott, J. and Kushner, S. (2007) 'The Need for a Manifesto for Educational Programme Evaluation', in *Cambridge Journal of Education*, Vol. 37(3), pp. 321–336

Estrella, M. (2000) 'Learning from Change', in M. Estrella (ed.), *Learning From Change: Issues and Experiences in Participatory Monitoring and Evaluation*, London: Intermediate Technology Publications Ltd, pp. 1–14

Everitt, A. and Hardiker, P. (1996) *Evaluating for Good Practice*, Basingstoke: Palgrave

Fals-Borda, O. (ed.) (1998) *People's Participation: Challenges Ahead*, New York: The Apex Press

Fals-Borda, O. and Rahman, M. (1991) *Action and Knowledge: Breaking the Monopoly with Participatory Action Research*, New York: Intermediate Technology Pubs/Apex Pres

Fetterman, D. and Wandersman, A. (2007) 'Empowerment Evaluation: Yesterday, Today and Tomorrow', in *American Journal of Evaluation*, Vol. 28(2), pp. 179–198

Fitzsimons, A., Hope, M., Russell, K. and Cooper, C. (2011) *Empowerment and Participation in Youth Work*, Exeter: Learning Matters

Foucault, M. (1975) *Discipline and Punish*, London: Allen Lane

Freire, P. (1970) *Pedagogy of the Oppressed*, London: Penguin

Froggett, L. (2002) *Love, Hate and Welfare*, Bristol: The Policy Press

Giddens, A. (1984) *The Constitution of Society: Outline of the Theory of Structuration*, Cambridge: Polity Press

Graham, K. and Harris, A. (2005) 'New Deal for Communities as a Participatory Public Policy: The Challenges for Evaluation', in D. Taylor and S. Balloch (eds), *The Politics of Evaluation*, Bristol: The Policy Press, pp. 97–108

Gregory, A. (2000) 'Problematizing Participation: A Critical Review of Approaches to Participation in Evaluation Theory', in *Evaluation*, Vol. 6(2), pp. 179–199

Groundwater-Smith, S., Dockett, S. and Bottrell, D. (2015) *Participatory Research with Children and Young People*, London: Sage Publications

Guba, E. and Lincoln, Y. (1989) *Fourth Generation Evaluation*, London: Sage Publications

Guijt, I. (2014) Participatory Approaches, Methodological Briefs: Impact Evaluation 5, UNICEF: Florence, accessed at www.unicef-irc.org/publications/750 (15.03.16)

Guijt, I. and Gaventa, J. (1998) Participatory Monitoring and Evaluation, IDS Policy Briefing 12, Brighton: Institute of Development Studies, accessed at www.ids.ac.uk/files/dmfile/PB12.pdf (10.03.16)

Hart, R. (1992) *Children's Participation: From Tokenism to Citizenship*, Florence: UNICEF, accessed at www.unicef-irc.org/publications/pdf/childrens_participation.pdf (10.03.16)

Hill, M., Davis, J., Prout, A. and Tisdall, K. (2004) 'Moving the Participation Agenda Forward', in *Children & Society*, Vol. 18(2), pp. 77–96

Issitt, M. and Spence, J. (2005) 'Practitioner Knowledge and Evidence-based Research, Policy and Practice', in *Youth & Policy*, Vol. 88, pp. 63–82

Jackson, E. and Kassam, Y. (eds) (1998) *Knowledge Shared: Participatory Evaluation in Development Cooperation*, Boulder, CO: Kumarian Press/IDRC

Jeffrey, L. (2011) *Understanding Agency: Social Welfare and Social Change*, Bristol: The Policy Press

Kemshall, H. and Littlechild, R. (eds) (2000) *User Involvement and Participation in Social Care*, London: Jessica Kingsley Publishers Ltd

Lansdown, G. (2005) Can You Hear Me? The Right of Young Children to Participate in Decisions Affecting Them. Working Paper 36. Bernard van Leer Foundation, The Hague, The Netherlands, accessed at http://resourcecentre.savethechildren.se/sites/default/files/documents/1235.pdf (10.03.16)

Ledwith, M. and Springett, J. (2010) *Participatory Practice: Community-based Action for Transformative Change*, Bristol: The Policy Press

Maguire, P. (1987) *Doing Participatory Research: A Feminist Approach*, Amherst, MA: Center for International Education

Mullender, A., Ward, D. and Fleming, J. (2013) *Empowerment in Action*, Basingstoke: Palgrave Macmillan

Mullinix, B. and Akalsa-Bukachi, M. (1998) 'Participatory Evaluation: Offering Kenyan Women Power and Voice', in E. Jackson and Y. Kassam (eds), *Knowledge Shared: Participatory Evaluation in Development Cooperation*, Boulder, CO: Kumarian Press, pp. 167–176

Ord, J. (2007) *Youth Work Process, Product and Practice*, Lyme Regis: Russell House Publishing

Reason, P. (1994) 'Three Approaches to Participative Inquiry', in N. Denzin and Y. Lincoln (eds), *Handbook of Qualitative Research*, London: Sage Publications, pp. 324–339

Ryan, K. (1998) 'Advantages and Challenges of Using Inclusive Evaluation Approaches in Evaluation Practice', in *American Journal of Evaluation*, Vol. 19(1), pp. 101–122

Sillitoe, P. (2002) 'Participatory Observation to Participatory Development: Making Anthropology Work', in P. Sillitoe, A. Bicker and J. Pottier (eds), *Participating in Development: Approaches to Indigenous Knowledge*, London: Routledge, pp. 1–23

Smith, M. (2001) 'Evaluation: Theory and Practice', *Encyclopaedia of Informal Education*, accessed at www.infed.org (12.01.17)

Suárez-Herrera, J., Springett, J. and Kagan, C. (2009) 'Critical Connections between Participatory Evaluation, Organizational Learning and Intentional Change in Pluralistic Organizations', in *Evaluation*, Vol. 15(3), pp. 321–342

Toal, S. (2009) 'The Validation of the Evaluation Involvement Scale for Use in Multisite Settings', in *American Journal of Evaluation*, Vol. 30(3), pp. 349–362

Treseder, P. (1997) *Empowering Children and Young People: Training Manual*, London: Save the Children

United Nations High Commission for Human Rights (1989) *Convention on the Rights of the Child*, Geneva: Office of the United Nations

White, S., Sadanandan Nair, K. and Ashcroft, J. (eds) (1994) *Participatory Communication: Working for Change and Development*, London: Sage Publications

Whitmore, E. (1991) 'Evaluation and Empowerment: It's the Process that Counts', in *Empowerment and Family Support Networking Bulletin*, Vol. 2(2), pp. 1–7

5

PARTICIPATORY EVALUATION APPROACHES

Introduction

The growth in the range of participatory approaches over the past four decades coincides with an increased interest in developing evaluation capacity (Labin, Duffy, Meyers, Wandersman and Lesesne 2012). This chapter explores three participatory evaluation approaches that centralise the position of stakeholders. These approaches, empowerment evaluation, collaborative evaluation and democratic evaluation, have been chosen as they reflect, to varying extents, the ethos and values of youth and community work, namely participation, inclusion, empowerment and social justice. The chapter begins with a brief discussion of similarities and distinguishing features. This is followed by an in-depth consideration of each approach, documenting their origins, developments and underlying principles. Practice examples of the three approaches are presented to illustrate how these forms of participatory evaluation can be used. The concluding section considers the critiques raised in relation to evaluation approaches that foreground stakeholder involvement.

Similarities and distinguishing features

The three approaches examined in this chapter (empowerment evaluation, collaborative evaluation and democratic evaluation) share a common aim of increasing stakeholder involvement. The purpose of this is to increase commitment and consequently evaluation use and influence, and to develop local evaluation capacity (Smith 2007). The essential processes of negotiation and relationship building are seen across these approaches, as is the belief that the complexities of context are best understood through dialogue and deliberation between evaluators and stakeholder communities. Drawing on Whitmore, Guijt, Mertens, Imm, Chinman and Wandersman (2006), empowerment evaluation, collaborative evaluation and democratic evaluation share four common underpinning principles (see Table 5.1).

TABLE 5.1 Common principles of participatory approaches

Participation	Multiple perspectives and experiences are recognised and valued. Importance is placed on democratic inclusion. Questions are asked as to who initiates and who drives evaluation and whose perspectives are emphasised.
Learning	Focus is placed on practical or action-orientated learning, and learning is both seen as an individual and collective process. Importance is given to the creation of a learning culture on the assumption that this leads to enhanced accountability as participants feel more responsible for what happens.
Negotiation	Fostering dialogue and deliberation enables negotiation of meanings, perspectives, roles and responsibilities and contributes to a sense of shared ownership which is seen as essential for sustained impact.
Flexibility	There is an understanding that the process of 'working together' is continually evolving and requires tolerance of ambiguity. The process is often characterised as cyclical and multilayered.

Cousins and Shulha (2006) identify five dimensions of stakeholder involvement:

- who controls decision making;
- diversity among stakeholders;
- the power relations between participating stakeholders;
- manageability of the evaluation implementation; and
- depth of participation.

Importantly, the three approaches under review in this chapter all accept that the range of stakeholders and the depth of their participation can vary depending on the specific evaluation.

Whether these approaches are, or indeed should be distinct from one another has been a long-running debate. Cousins, Whitmore and Shulha (2012) state their preference to use the term 'collaborative evaluation' as an umbrella term that encompasses a number of approaches including empowerment evaluation and democratic evaluation. They argue that attempts to compartmentalise different forms of participatory evaluation is unwarranted and unproductive, particularly in terms of advancing thinking about theory and practice.

On the other side of the debate, Fetterman, Rodríguez-Campos, Wandersman and O'Sullivan (2014: 144) argue that: 'defining, compartmentalising and differentiating among stakeholder approaches to evaluation, (....) enhances conceptual clarity. It also informs practice, helping evaluators select the most appropriate approach for the task at hand.' For them, the distinction rests on who is in control of the evaluation; for example, they propose that in collaborative evaluation, the evaluator is in charge, whereas in empowerment evaluation, it is the stakeholders who are in control. Instead, Fetterman et al. (2014) propose 'stakeholder involvement approaches' as a more appropriate umbrella term. In the next section, empowerment evaluation, collaborative evaluation and democratic evaluation are examined in detail, offering the reader the opportunity to decide on whether or not these approaches are distinct or not.

Empowerment evaluation

Fetterman developed the empowerment evaluation approach in the 1990s in the USA. He defined empowerment evaluation as 'the use of evaluation concepts, techniques and findings to foster improvement and self determination' (Fetterman 2001: 3). Empowerment evaluation is an appropriate evaluation approach when the primary goal is to actively engage programme participants and staff in the evaluation process. The emphasis on fostering self determination was, at that time, what set it apart from other approaches (Patton 2005).

For some this shift in thinking was problematic; for example, Stufflebeam (1994) argued that empowerment evaluation confused the purpose of evaluation. He viewed the purpose to be the systematic assessment of merit or worth, not the achievement of self-determination. Fetterman defended his position, arguing that the investigation of worth or merit and plans for programme improvement are the means through which self-determination can be actualised.

Empowerment evaluation positions assessment of worth as secondary to social change. The definition of empowerment evaluation has developed over time and is now seen as:

> An evaluation approach that aims to increase the probability of achieving program success by
>
> 1. providing program stakeholders with tools for assessing the planning, implementation, and self-evaluation of their program, and
> 2. mainstreaming evaluation as part of the planning and management of the program/organization. (Wandersman, Snell-Johns, Lentz, Fetterman, Keener, Livet, Imm and Flaspohler 2005: 28)

A set of ten principles which underpin empowerment evaluation were offered alongside this new definition (see Table 5.2).

Some have questioned the lack of reference to self-determination in this new definition of empowerment evaluation. Miller and Campbell (2006) point to the absence of the language of liberation, empowerment, and transformation, arguing that this has been replaced by an emphasis on capacity building and sustained evaluative thinking in organisations. Patton (2005) also notes the absence of self-determination as a principle, but concluded that 'the definition of empowerment evaluation as centering on self determination remains unchanged' (ibid.: 409). Fetterman and Wandersman (2007) accept that the new definition has an emphasis on programme success and state that this definition does not replace the original, 'it provides more of an elaboration than a substitution' (ibid.: 186).

TABLE 5.2 The principles of empowerment evaluation (from Wandersman et al. 2005: 30)

Principle 1	Improvement
Principle 2	Community ownership
Principle 3	Inclusion
Principle 4	Democratic participation
Principle 5	Social justice
Principle 6	Community knowledge
Principle 7	Evidence-based strategies
Principle 8	Capacity-building
Principle 9	Organisational learning
Principle 10	Accountability

Wandersman and Snell-Johns (2005: 422) assert that 'empowerment evaluation is not defined by its methods but by the collaborative manner in which methods are applied according to the empowerment evaluation principles'. In a review of forty seven case examples, Miller and Campbell (2006) identified three modes of empowerment evaluation practice as follows:

Socratic coaching	The evaluator maintains a question-and-answer relationship with stakeholders to promote the development of the evaluative knowledge. A facilitative role is taken in supporting the group to collectively agree on evaluation aims, design and procedures, and to collect, analyse and report evaluation data.
Structured guidance	The evaluator typically designs the process of evaluation, and provides guidance for stakeholders in the form of manuals or templates and stakeholders develop their evaluative knowledge through use. Analysis and reporting is often conducted by the evaluator.
Participatory evaluation	The evaluator designs and implements the study. Stakeholders provide feedback on elements and/or participate in pre-defined areas. For example, this may include offering advice on recruiting respondents or helping with data collection.

Miller and Campbell (2006) argue that while empowerment evaluation was originally framed as an approach that benefitted a wide range of stakeholders, the way in which it was practiced benefitted a much narrower group. Essentially those who benefit are those who run or deliver programmes:

The goal of empowering citizens who are the beneficiaries of social programs has become less salient in cases of empowerment evaluation practice than has increasing the self determining status of program staff members and managers and holding the program staff members accountable to funding institutions. (Miller and Campbell 2006: 314)

Significant differences were found when assessing the extent to which these different modes enacted the principles of empowerment evaluation. The Socratic coaching mode was seen to hold the majority of the principles to some extent, particularly in relation to organisational learning, inclusion, social justice and democracy. In stark contrast, none of the forty-seven cases classified as 'structured guidance' evidenced social justice or democratic principles. In this mode it was accountability that was most evident.

Empowerment evaluation in practice

It is the way in which the principles of empowerment evaluation are applied that shapes its practice. The particular evaluation methods used are likely to be determined by a range of factors, for example, the purpose of the evaluation, what is being evaluated, and the resources available to conduct the evaluation. The evaluation methods used in an empowerment evaluation are often similar to those used in other forms of participatory evaluation. While there are no specific steps that must be followed within empowerment evaluation, there are a number of models that can be used to inform an organisation as to how they might use an empowerment evaluation approach. Here we will look at two, both of which were developed in the USA.

The first model comes from CDC's (1999) 'Framework for Program Evaluation in Public Health'. This model contains six steps as shown in Table 5.3.

TABLE 5.3 CDC's (1999) 'Framework for Program Evaluation in Public Health'

Step	Action	Description
1	Engage stakeholders	This includes staff, those in receipt of or affected by the program and the primary users of the evaluation.
2	Describe the program strategy	Articulate the need, expected effects, activities, resources, stage, context and logic model for the program.
3	Focus the evaluation design	Assess the issues of greatest concern to stakeholders. Consider the purpose, users, questions, methods and agreements, and effective use of time.
4	Gather credible evidence	This involves generating information that stakeholders perceive as trustworthy and relevant to addresses their questions. Evidence can be experimental or observational, qualitative or quantitative, or it can include a mixture of methods.
5	Justify conclusions	This involves linking conclusions to the evidence gathered and judging them against agreed-upon values or standards set by the stakeholders. Use five elements to justify conclusions: standards, analysis/synthesis, interpretation, judgement and recommendations.
6	Ensure use (findings use and process use)	It is important that stakeholders are aware of the evaluation findings and that the findings are considered in decisions or actions that affect the program. Equally it is important that those who participated in the evaluation process have had a beneficial experience.

The second model is the 'Getting to Outcomes' model. This ten-step approach was specifically designed for organisations whose aim is to prevent or reduce drug and tobacco use among young people (Chinman, Imm and Wandersman 2004). The model is based on addressing ten accountability questions:

1. What are the underlying needs and conditions in the community? (Needs/Resources)
2. What are the goals, target populations, and objectives (i.e. desired outcomes)? (Goals)
3. Which evidence-based models and best practice programs can be useful in reaching the goals? (Best Practice)
4. What actions need to be taken so the selected program 'fits' the community context? (Fit)
5. What organizational capacities are needed to implement the plan? (Capacities)
6. What is the plan for this program? (Plan)
7. How will the quality of program and/or initiative implementation be assessed? (Process Evaluation)
8. How well did the program work? (Outcome Evaluation)
9. How will continuous quality improvement strategies be incorporated? (Continuous Quality Improvement)
10. If the program is successful, how will it be sustained? (Sustain)

(taken from Chinman, Imm and Wandersman 2004: 2)

This model combines traditional evaluation, empowerment evaluation, results-based accountability, and continuous quality improvement and aims to enhance practitioners' practice skills and empower them to plan, implement, and evaluate their own programmes.

Both models fall into the 'structured guidance' mode, the most prevalent mode in the review of empowerment evaluation case examples. This mode is generally used in large multi-site evaluations (Miller and Campbell 2006). Both models provide a set of steps designed in advance, however, they are described as examples of 'best practice process' in that while they are prescriptive, they are sufficiently flexible to be used in any change-orientated programme.

There is an interesting shift in discourse between these two models, particularly in regards to accountability, for example, the Getting to Outcomes model is based on addressing accountability questions. Arguably, these questions do not necessarily require the inclusion of service-users or promote democratic principles.

This may be an unavoidable consequence of the complexity of conducting large-scale, multi-site evaluations; equally it may reflect the strengthening of the discourse of accountability during this time period. Miller and Campbell (2006) call for a re-examination of the ten principles of empowerment evaluation and for an analysis of how to implement these principles in practice. Smith (2007) rightly questions whether self-determination and empowerment can really remain as the defining characteristics of empowerment evaluation. Fetterman and Wandersman (2007: 186) respond to this challenge by stating that 'self determination is basic to empowerment evaluation and will continue to be a central part of the definition of empowerment evaluation'.

Collaborative evaluation

Collaborative approaches in evaluation have become increasing popular, particularly in cross-cultural contexts where they are considered better suited than more traditional approaches. There are a number of benefits associated with collaborative evaluation. Firstly, because programme staff are actively engaged in the design of the evaluation it is considered that it will reflect a more accurate understanding of the programme and the concerns of stakeholders. Weiss (1998: 25) highlights the 'process use' element of collaborative evaluation (see Chapter 7 for a more detailed discussion of process use). She states it is:

> helping program people reflect on their practice, think critically, and ask questions about why the program operates as it does. They learn something of the evaluative cast of mind—the sceptical questioning point of view, the perspective of the reflective practitioner (ibid.: 25)

Rodríguez-Campos (2012) argues that stakeholders are also more likely to understand and use evaluation findings because they participated in framing the evaluation design and process from the beginning.

However, there is no universally agreed definition as to what collaborative evaluation is, indeed there is differing opinion as to whether it should be considered as a distinct theoretical model or as an umbrella term. Cousins et al. (2012) argue the latter, voicing concerns that collaborative evaluations need to be principle-driven, rather than model- or method-driven. For them, there is not a distinct model; they view collaborative evaluation as an approach that includes multiple forms of evaluation. In contrast, O'Sullivan (2004) distinguishes collaborative evaluation from participatory evaluation and empowerment evaluation. She does this on the basis that, in her view, participatory evaluation does not always require stakeholder decision-making in the evaluation process and empowerment evaluation has participant empowerment as a direct outcome of the evaluation process, which is not the case for collaborative evaluation. O'Sullivan (2004: 26) argues:

> Collaborative evaluation is often empowering to participants. It enhances their understanding of evaluation so that they gain new skills. As such it [empowerment] is a valuable outcome of the process, but not as an intended outcome as described by Fetterman et al. (1996) or Burke (1998).

She asserts that it is the emphasis on stakeholder engagement at each stage of the evaluation that distinguishes collaborative evaluation from other forms of participatory evaluation.

Rodríguez-Campos and Rincones-Gómez (2013: 4) view collaborative evaluation as: 'An evaluation in which there is a substantial degree of collaboration between evaluators and stakeholders in the evaluation process, to the extent that they are willing and capable of being involved.' They note that ongoing discussions within the American Evaluation Association's Collaborative, Participative and Empowerment Evaluation Topical Interest Group have resulted in a 'cautiously developed definition' of collaborative evaluation, expressed in terms of the role of the evaluator:

> Collaborative evaluators are in charge of the evaluation, but they create an ongoing engagement between evaluators and stakeholders, contributing to stronger evaluation designs, enhanced data collection and analysis, and results that stakeholders understand and use. (Rodríguez-Campos and O'Sullivan [2010] cited in Rodríguez-Campos and Rincones-Gómez [2013: 2])

Accepting this consensus definition of collaborative evaluation, it is important to note the determination of leadership and decision-making responsibility is dependent on the particular evaluation situation. It is necessary to take account of a number of factors, including the evaluation culture within the organisation, previous evaluation experiences and the organisational climate, when determining the possible level of collaboration (O'Sullivan 2004).

Collaborative evaluation does not require all stakeholders to participate in every evaluation activity, but it does require that decisions about roles are made explicit and that these are based on the feasibility, time, skills and interest of stakeholders to participate in each phase. Cousins et al. (2012) make the point that collaboration needs to be negotiated between evaluators and stakeholders if it is to be meaningful, productive and beneficial for those involved. This process of negotiation is essential and ongoing, and it is through dialogue and deliberation that the complexities of each particular context are understood. It is this process that shapes the evaluation and enables decision-making in regards to deciding control, and the diversity and level of participation.

Rodríguez-Campos (2005) identified seven 'collaboration guiding principles' which she claimed represented the diversity of perceptions in regards to the primary purpose of collaboration. These principles: (a) development, (b) empowerment, (c) involvement, (d) qualification, (e) social support, (f) trust, and (g) understanding, are presented as general ideals or expectations that needed to be considered when engaging in collaborative evaluation. The principles were re-stated in 2013 (Rodríguez-Campos and Rincones-Gómez 2013) with only minor changes, so it seems they have stood the test of time. The order in which they are presented changed from 2005 to 2013 with the principle 'understanding' being re-named as 'empathy' and coming second in the list presented in 2013. However, this re-positioning may be insignificant as the list is presented, in both publications, as an integrated one which implies no hierarchy. The seven principles presented in 2013 are summarised in Table 5.4.

Shulha, Whitmore, Cousins, Gilbert and Hudib (2016) engaged in a four-year empirical study to develop an integrated set of eight evidenced-based principles to guide

TABLE 5.4 Collaboration guiding principles (from Rodríguez-Campos and Rincones-Gómez 2013: 179–181)

Development	This principle calls for an appreciation of different learning styles and for these to be addressed according to the particular situation. It also implies a commitment to continuously seeking to improve collaborative opportunities and a shared responsibility to contribute to each other's learning and an avoidance of inadequate actions that detract from each other's development.
Empathy	This principle implies that sensitive and/or uncomfortable topics are acknowledged and dealt with in a sensitive, understanding and thoughtful way. Personal perspectives and biases are identified and explored to enable a full understanding. It implies a commitment to creating a safe and open environment for discussion in which views can be expressed especially when these differ.
Empowerment	This principle implies everyone has responsibilities and authority to make decisions on specific tasks and accountability for subsequent results. It involves a commitment to enabling a sense of self-efficacy by delegating authority and removing obstacles that may limit achievement.
Involvement	This principle involves actively engaging everyone in making decisions and taking action by recognising the need to take joint actions for a mutual cause.
Qualification	This principle implies a responsibility for maintaining the personal and professional qualifications needed.
Social support	This principle implies that obtaining support from a broad range of people is central to collaborative work and that the prevention of conflicts of interest as a result of the collaboration is everyone's responsibility.
Trust	This principle implies that a high level of mutual trust enables collaboration.

those looking to use collaborative evaluation in practice. They suggest that the value of the principles is twofold: firstly, in their capacity to illuminate complexity rather than resolve it, and secondly, in their capacity to inform decisions rather than prescribe them. There is a degree of caution shown by the authors:

> We make no claims that this set as it stands today is either exhaustive or enduring (...) we introduce a set of empirically grounded principles that individually, and as a set, show promise in guiding evaluation practice in contexts where the meaning of evaluation is jointly constructed by evaluators and stakeholders. (Shulha et al. 2016: 196)

The principles are as follows:

- clarify motivation for collaboration;
- foster meaningful relationships;

- develop a shared understanding of the programme;
- promote appropriate participatory processes;
- monitor and respond to the resource availability;
- monitor evaluation progress and quality;
- promote evaluative thinking;
- follow through to realise use.

While each principle is seen as being essential, the importance given to any particular principle is dependent on contextual conditions, circumstance and the degree of complexity. In order for these principles to be relevant, they need to demonstrate their potential to strengthen collaborations. Shulha et al. (2016) assert that the interdependence of the principles need to be made explicit, and acknowledge that the value of these principles rests with the extent to which they are able to add value to collaborative work and enhance evaluators' practice knowledge.

Collaborative evaluation in practice

Three different models, developed in practice, will be discussed. The first is a simple five-stage model designed by Brackett and Hurley (2004) for use by education practitioners with limited evaluation knowledge or experience. The model seeks to promote reflection and learning among practitioners and to be led by them in their own learning communities. It involves an ongoing process with each cycle having five stages as shown in Figure 5.1.

Brackett and Hurley (2004) identify a threefold purpose of collaborative evaluation. Firstly, it supports the continuous assessment of progress to inform programme improvement at the district, school, and classroom levels. Secondly, it enables the development of authentic and relevant documentation for use with a variety of audiences, especially present and future funders. Lastly, the engagement of stakeholders in the evaluation supports evaluation capacity building at a local level and the development of learning communities. The simplicity of the model is particularly valuable as it provides an accessible guide for anyone new to collaborative evaluation; it is transferable to other contexts and appropriate for small-scale projects in terms of resource requirements.

The second model is more complex. Rodríguez-Campos and Rincones-Gómez (2013), drawing on their experiences of collaborative work in the business, non-profit and education sectors present a Model for Collaborative Evaluations (MCE). This is a detailed model that consists of six interactive components that are aligned with particular stages of the evaluation. Each component has up to five subcomponents (see Figure 5.2), all of which are supported by a ten-step guide to support understanding.

Rodríguez-Campos and Rincones-Gómez are keen to point out that, although the model could be seen to promote an expectation of a sequential process, it should be interpreted more as a system, where continuous review and feedback bring

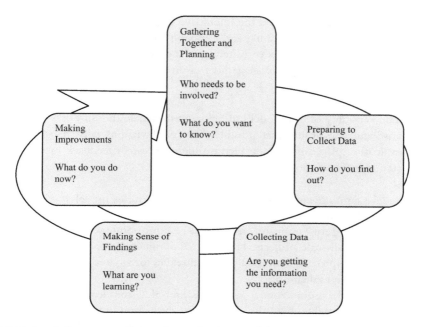

FIGURE 5.1 A five-stage collaborative evaluation model

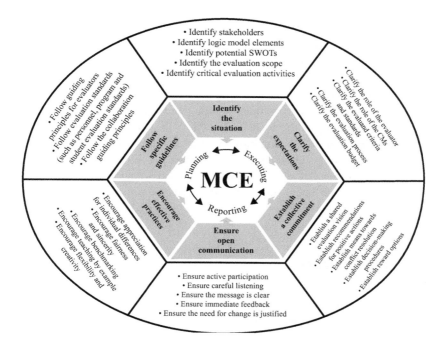

FIGURE 5.2 Model for Collaborative Evaluations (MCE) (Rodríguez-Campos and Rincones-Gómez 2013: 6)

about change. They recommend the interactive use of the elements (components and subcomponents) on a 'rotating and remixing basis'. The model also provides an iterative checklist that offers consistent guidance and the feedback mechanisms support the identification and management of unanticipated or unintended events during the evaluation:

> The versatility of this model can help you to handle the 'surprises' that may arise and also ensure that possible flaws or deviations with regard to the evaluation plan can be controlled through the use of feedback mechanisms (Rodríguez-Campos and Rincones-Gómez 2013: 7)

This model is far more complex than the Brackett and Hurley model. It will require a greater level of understanding from the outset, and as such, it may need to be facilitated by an external evaluator. It may also be more complex than necessary for evaluation of small-scale projects. However, Rodríguez-Campos and Rincones-Gómez (2013) do provide a succinct set of guidelines for anyone looking to implement collaborative evaluation.

The third model is not a model per se, it is a set of 'lessons learned' that provide some interesting insights about the collaborative evaluation in practice. Corn et al. (2012) conducted a study of the experiences of those involved in collaborative evaluation within the field of education in North Carolina. They present their findings as a series of 'lessons learned' and offer suggestions in response. Their nine lessons are summarised in Table 5.5.

Corn, Byrom, Knestis, Matzen and Thrift (2012) draw two important conclusions from their study; firstly they note that evaluation capacity building requires a significant amount of time, energy, and resources and that while support and guidance from an external evaluator is beneficial, the difference is made when that person has a comprehensive understanding and appreciation of the context. Their second point is that the focus of the effort should be on the practitioners and their projects, not on learning how to do evaluation. They argue that collaborative evaluation is not 'about project evaluation per se; it is about supporting the underlying purpose of the evaluation – educators having solid information and tools they can use in making sound decisions for improving their projects, which translates into more effective teaching and improved outcomes for students' (Corn et al. 2012: 14).

Democratic evaluation

Democratic evaluation was developed in the late 1970s and early 1980s and sought to promote democratic processes, institutions and participation. Its foundations lie with the work of Barry MacDonald in England and Ernest House in North America. MacDonald (1976) provided the original formulation of democratic evaluation and put forward a heuristic framework of macro politics and micro relationships. He argued the macro positioning of

TABLE 5.5 Lessons learned about collaborative evaluation (from Corn et al. 2012)

Lesson	Suggested action
Different stakeholder groups see different purposes for the evaluation of educational programs and projects.	• Recognise that learning how to use evaluation data is more important than learning how to develop and implement plans. • Provide feedback to stakeholders based on data collected.
Language matters.	• Early in the project, establish and maintain a "team glossary," created by the group responsible for managing the project and its evaluation.
It's important for all of the players in an evaluation to understand each other's roles.	• Clarify the roles and responsibilities of all individuals participating in evaluation activities at all levels, and have a plan for making sure that they are understood by all involved.
The time that teachers have for working on a project evaluation is limited.	• Use time that has already been dedicated for planning and decision making activities, such as staff meetings, for completing surveys, reflective journals, activity checklists, or other data-collection instruments.
Developing the capacity for formative evaluation can change not only projects, but also the people implementing the projects.	• Have a framework for monitoring, thinking about, and discussing the changes the stakeholders and their projects were going through.
In developing the capacity for formative evaluation, teachers and administrators do not need to become evaluation experts, but they do need to develop specific evaluation skills.	• Rather than adding a lot of new data collection procedures, try making simple adjustments to data already being collected.
Success in implementing a project evaluation—and likely of the project itself—depends in large measure on participants sharing a sense of identity around both the project and the valuation.	• If logic-mapping strategies are thought to be valuable, apply them early in the project planning process and with enough flexibility that planning teams can illustrate their collective understanding of how their project works. • Develop a plan to actively share project and evaluation plans, activities, and results with stakeholders.
Communication is the glue that holds a project evaluation together.	• Set aside time early in the project, for the team and staff to discuss the best ways of communicating and to ensure that communication is meaningful and timely.
One size evaluation does not fit all.	• Before asking an organisation to adopt new approaches, find out what is working, what the constraints might be and what evaluation efforts they are able to take on; then provide evaluation support to meet their needs.

evaluation allowed questions to be asked about the purpose of evaluation and about whose interest should be served. Micro relationships focus on the relationships between evaluators and stakeholders and the processes and interactions that shape those relationships. He saw democratic evaluation as a means of legitimising multiple stakeholders' perspectives and serving the public's right to know (Greene 2006).

MacDonald was explicit about the political nature of evaluation stating 'Evaluators not only live in the real world of educational politics: they actually influence its changing power relationships' (MacDonald 1976: 125). He proposed a typology of evaluation based on political classification: bureaucratic, autocratic and democratic. The first two, bureaucratic evaluation and autocratic evaluation both serve government agencies that are already empowered to allocate resources and determine policy direction. The former is an unconditional service in which the evaluator acts in the role of consultant; their work is neither independent nor available for public scrutiny. The latter, autocratic evaluation, is a conditional service in which the evaluator retains independence and ownership of results which are validated by the evaluation community.

The third classification, democratic evaluation, serves the public interest in addition to the established interests of policymakers. The methods involved and results gained, are presented in ways that are accessible to non-specialists and all participants have control over the form and release of the evaluation results. MacDonald set out to broaden the scope of evaluation in terms of the questions it addressed and thus the interests served. He also sought to increase the range of people in receipt of evaluation findings in order to enable public engagement in informed discussions about policy issues and directions. In other words, he wanted to democratise knowledge in evaluation. As such, he saw evaluation as a means to critique policy. In essence, democratic evaluation requires evaluators to act democratically particularly in regards to the control of, access to and release of evaluation findings.

House and Howe (1999) developed the deliberative democratic approach to evaluation, the aims of which are to:

- represent a wide range of views and interests in evaluation studies;
- encourage stakeholder participation in evaluation processes;
- provide opportunities for extended deliberation.

Deliberative democratic evaluation is characterised by three principles; liberation, inclusion and dialogue. Evaluations taking this approach seek to contribute to advancing democracy in a democratic society (Ryan 2005). Deliberation in this context is seen as 'reasoning reflectively about relevant issues, including identifying preferences and values of all stakeholder groups' (Ryan 2005: 2). Deliberative democratic evaluation is by nature dialogical and it is argued that it is through dialogue that stakeholder interests, opinions and ideas can be more accurately and more completely portrayed.

There is not a prescribed method or model of democratic evaluation; however, House and Howe (1999: 113) offered ten guiding questions for evaluators using this approach. These are:

1. Whose interests are represented?
2. Are major stakeholders represented?
3. Are any major stakeholders excluded?
4. Are there serious power imbalances?
5. Are there procedures to control power imbalances?
6. How do people participate in the evaluation?
7. How authentic is their interaction?
8. How involved is their interaction?
9. Is there reflective deliberation?
10. How considered and extensive is the deliberation?

McTaggart (1991) questioned how democratic some democratic evaluations were, arguing that a clear distinction between representative and participatory democracy is needed. For him, democratic evaluations need to embrace participatory democracy to include the voice of all stakeholders if they are to enhance citizens' interest in politics and democracy and champion issues that are neglected or not sufficiently covered by the elected representatives. He recognises that:

> Reconceptualising evaluation in participatory [democracy] terms clearly would not remove the possibility of conflict between site participants, but it would give them a chance to negotiate among themselves forms of knowledge production which enhanced the possibilities for their work. (McTaggart 1991: 20)

Cockburn (2010) identifies three broad forms of democracy that have informed work in relation to young people's participation in England, these are summarised in Table 5.6.

The three interrelated principles that inform democratic evaluation are inclusion, dialogue, and deliberation (House and Howe 1999). The principle of

TABLE 5.6 Three forms of democracy (from Cockburn 2010)

Representational democracy	This form involves the model of an identified (elected) person to represent the views of a much larger group in decision-making.
Participatory democracy	This form emphasises the involvement of everyone in decision-making and involves the democratisation of everyday life.
Deliberative democracy	This form lies somewhere between the two and involves a selection to represent the population. Those selected are not necessarily 'elected'; they may be selected randomly using a structured sample design.

inclusion necessitates that all groups with a significant interest in the evaluation be included. The degree of inclusion may vary from evaluation to evaluation in terms of how, and at which stage, people are included and will be dependent on the existent background knowledge, the nature of the questions to be addressed, the available resources and the timescale. However, inclusivity alone is no guarantee of democracy, particularly when inclusion is passive. Howe and Ashcraft (2005: 2276) argue that 'Passive inclusion is not enough to ensure that the voices included will be genuine. This requires active inclusion, which shades into the requirement of dialogue.' They identify two forms of dialogue; elucidating and critical. For them, elucidating dialogue is limited to clarifying participants' views and self-understandings whereas critical dialogue includes both clarifying and scrutinising these views and self-understandings. It is this form of dialogue that underpins democratic evaluation.

Democratic evaluation has been implemented successfully for four decades (Ryan 2004) and has significant advantages. For example, the evaluation is grounded in the experiences and viewpoints of the stakeholders who come together to validate the findings. Stakeholders' participation in the democratic process results in feedback that strengthens decision-making, planning and strategic development (Love and Muggah 2005). However, House and Howe (1999) explicitly acknowledged that deliberative democratic evaluation is an ideal, and some may argue that it is too idealised to be put directly into practice. In response, Howe and Ashcraft (2005) suggest that even partial implementation of this approach is helpful for enacting democratic processes and Greene (2006: 124) asserts 'the ideal can still serve us as a useful guide and framework for evaluation practice'.

Some identify the current evaluation discourse as a major challenge. For example, Weiss (2005) notes the peripheral position of democratic evaluation and Ryan (2004) acknowledges the challenges posed by dominance of an audit culture characterised by power and authority. She offers encouragement to those who support a more democratic approach by arguing that:

> this does not mean democratic approaches should not be practiced. Democratic evaluation is intended for contexts where there are concerns about top-down control of management and education (MacDonald and Kushner 2004). Further, democratic evaluation fits well when institutions are interested in moving to less hierarchical, more horizontal arrangements.
> (Ryan 2004: 456)

Democratic evaluation offers considerable promise, but for this to be realised Greene (2006: 136) tells us that as well as addressing the ideological challenges, the practical challenges also need to addressed, these include:

> Meaningfully operationalising lofty democratic ideals and commitments in specific contexts, developing facilitation and dialogical skills in evaluators, creating the time and space for messy processes like participation and

deliberation, and maintaining methodological excellence while advocating for democratic ideals.

Democratic evaluation in practice

While there is a growing literature base relating to democratic evaluation, there has not been a growth of models for practice. Arguably, this is because democratic evaluation is more about the evaluator's role, stance and value commitments than about particular methods or tools – this of course makes for challenging times when trying to put it into practice. House (2005) provides three examples of democratic evaluations that do help in terms of illuminating the variety of methods:

1. The first example took place in a social work context in Sweden. Stakeholder groups, involving politicians, practitioners, parents, and young people, were interviewed by an external evaluator. The interview findings from each group were then presented to each of the other groups, their reactions collected and presented to the others again. Representatives from all groups then came together to discuss the findings face-to-face, and the deliberations of the meetings formed part of the evaluation.
2. The second example is an evaluation of a court-ordered bilingual education programme conducted by House himself. Lawyers and school administrators were involved in both the evaluation design and the data collection. Preliminary findings were presented in face-to-face meetings bi-annually, providing the opportunity for the two groups to react to the findings and to each other, as well as to refocus the study as it progressed.
3. The third example comes from an educational research context, in Britain. In this example preliminary survey findings were sent to all participants who were then asked to respond whether they agreed with the findings and to give reasons where they did not agree. The conclusions in the final report were revised to take account of the deliberations.

A more recent example from practice is offered here in the form of a Deliberative Discussion Day (DDD), developed for use in a city in Finland in 2008 as a method to involve young people in the evaluation of the services provided for them (see Gretschel 2016). An important component of DDD is the aim to offer young people a channel for citizens' participation. Inclusion, good quality discussion and the connection to decision-making are considered central elements. The process begins with young people evaluating youth services in their area. As wide a range of young people's views as possible are sought. Young people in the locality who do not use the youth projects are contacted through other methods, for example, through street-based methods and through schools. A critical dialogue approach was taken in that young people were not only asked about the quality of provision but also asked whether the provision included the 'right' services. The youth workers and decision-makers evaluated the same services from perspectives identified and prioritised by the young people involved. The facilitators played a vital role in enabling a symmetrical relationship between the young people and the adults. This included having more young people than adults participating and young people being given more weight in terms of opportunities to speak.

Face-to-face discussions between young people and decision-makers are initiated by a statement, question or proposal prepared by the young people in advance. The results of the discussions are documented, reported and published, and a roadmap instrument is used to transform talk into action (Cooper and Gretschel, forthcoming). In this specific DDD example, the data produced were analysed for two purposes. Firstly, to identify the directions youth work should take and secondly, to shed new light on how and with which criteria the quality and accessibility of youth work provision should be reported at local and national levels.

The challenges associated with involving the stakeholder in evaluation

As stated earlier the common aspect of the three participatory approaches discussed in this chapter is the centrality of stakeholder engagement. There is much written about the benefits of involving a stakeholder, however, there is also a growing concern that stakeholder participation is not living up to many of the claims that are being made (Reed 2008). This final section highlights some of the challenges in implementing evaluation approaches that foreground stakeholder involvement.

The first, and perhaps most challenging, hurdle for those looking to work with stakeholders relates to values. It is highly likely that stakeholders will have multiple value orientations and these will inform their perceptions of a programme and of each other. Orr (2010) highlights further difficulties that may be encountered, for example, stakeholders may choose to focus on conflict more than on decision-making, there may be personal issues between participants, or there may be a lack of sufficient expertise or time to commit to the process.

Many of the challenges relate to issues of power. Stakeholder participation does not take place in a power vacuum. Cultural and contextual power differentials and dynamics need to be acknowledged and understood (Johnson 2010) if stakeholder engagement is to be meaningful. Organisational and professional power also need to be considered, as managerialist conceptions of accountability often restrict opportunities for shared control. Programme managers may have concerns about opening up decision-making to 'outside voices' due to fear of criticism or conflict, or worst, this may be driven by a reluctance to be transparent (Orr 2010). There are many ways in which stakeholder participation is enacted, and some forms of participation can reinforce existing power positions and group dynamics can restrict or discourage minority perspectives from being expressed creating what Cooke (2001: 19) terms 'dysfunctional consensus'.

Brandon and Fukunaga (2014) conducted a systematic review of forty-one peer-reviewed studies on stakeholder involvement in evaluation, and identified a range of issues that need to be addressed if stakeholder involvement is to realise its potential. Two related aspects stand out, namely resources and stakeholder selection. In relation to resources, evaluators who choose to adopt stakeholder involvement approaches will need enhanced interpersonal and leadership skills. Arguably, youth and community workers have these skills; engaging with a diverse range of people is what they do. As such, evaluation approaches that centralise stakeholder involvement should fit well in this context.

The stakeholders participating in the studies reviewed by Brandon and Fukunaga (2014) were mostly programme staff, and in many of the cases the number of participating stakeholders was small. This is perhaps indicative of the difficulties in maintaining consistent motivation and involvement over time and the amount of time that stakeholders need to commit when participating in evaluations. Involving a broad range of stakeholders in evaluations also requires a considerable staff time. Identifying, selecting, recruiting and maintaining stakeholders places additional demands on evaluators and programme staff.

Finally, evidencing the social justice effect of stakeholder involvement appears to be an even greater challenge. Studies highlight the absence of evidence that shows the effects of stakeholder involvement on social justice (Brandon and Fukunaga 2014; Miller and Campbell 2006). This is despite the fact that it is often cited as a primary purpose of some stakeholder involvement approaches. Clearly, social justice is a difficult and diffuse construct to measure as an effect of involving stakeholders, however, this does not mean that it should be written out. House (1980) argues that all evaluation methodologies embody assumptions about social justice as our methodological choices are informed by how we see the world. The challenge is to ensure we continually strive to move beyond rational decisions relating to the application of appropriate methods to the mobilisation of efforts that promote people's right to access to evaluation as a means of advancing social justice.

References

Brackett, A. and Hurley, N. (2004) Collaborative Evaluation Led by Local Educators: A Practical, Print- and Web-Based Guide, Northeast and the Islands Regional Technology in Education Consortium accessed at www.wested.org/resources/collaborative-evaluation-led-by-local-educators-a-practical-print-and-web-based-guide/ (21.07.16)

Brandon, P. and Fukunaga, L. (2014) 'The State of the Empirical Research Literature on Stakeholder Involvement in Program Evaluation', *American Journal of Evaluation*, Vol. 35(1), pp. 26–44

Centers for Disease Control and Prevention (CDC) (1999) 'Framework for Program Evaluation in Public Health', *Morbidity and Mortality Weekly Report*, 48 (RR-11), Atlanta, GA: Centers for Disease Control and Prevention

Chinman, M., Imm, P. and Wandersman, A. (2004) *Getting to Outcomes 2004: Promoting Accountability through Methods and Tools for Planning, Implementation, and Evaluation*, Santa Monica, CA: RAND Corporation.

Cockburn, T. (2010) 'Children and Deliberative Democracy in England', in B. Percy-Smith and N. Thomas (eds), *A Handbook of Children and Young People's Participation*, Abingdon: Routledge, pp. 306–317

Cooke, B. (2001) 'The Social Psychological Limits of Participation?', in B. Cooke and U. Kothari (eds), *Participation: The New Tyranny?* London: Zed Books, pp. 102–121

Cooper, S. and Gretschel, A. (forthcoming) 'Evaluating Youth Work in its Context', in *The Sage Handbook of Youth Work*, London: Sage Publications

Corn, J., Byrom, E., Knestis, K., Matzen, N. and Thrift, B. (2012) 'Lessons Learned About Collaborative Evaluation using the Capacity for Applying Project Evaluation (CAPE) Framework with School and District Leaders', *Evaluation and Program Planning*, Vol. 35(4), pp. 535–542

Cousins, J.B. and Shulha, L. (2006) 'A Comparative Analysis of Evaluation Utilization and its Cognate Fields of Enquiry: Current Issues and Trends', in I. Shaw, J. Greene and M. Mark (eds), *The Sage Handbook of Evaluation*, London: Sage Publications, pp. 266–291

Cousins, J.B., Whitmore, E. and Shulha, L. (2012) 'Arguments for a Common Set of Principles for Collaborative Inquiry in Evaluation', *American Journal of Evaluation*, Vol. 34(1), pp. 7–22

Fetterman, D. (2001) 'The Transformation of Evaluation into a Collaboration: A Vision of Evaluation in the 21st Century', *American Journal of Evaluation*, Vol. 22(3), pp. 381–385

Fetterman, D. and Wandersman, A. (2007) 'Empowerment Evaluation Yesterday, Today, and Tomorrow', *American Journal of Evaluation*, Vol. 28(2), pp. 179–198

Fetterman, D., Rodríguez-Campos, L., Wandersman, A. and O'Sullivan, R. (2014) 'Collaborative, Participatory, and Empowerment Evaluation: Building a Strong Conceptual Foundation for Stakeholder Involvement Approaches to Evaluation (A Response to Cousins, Whitmore, and Shulha 2013)', *American Journal of Evaluation*, Vol. 35(1), pp. 144–148

Greene, J. (2006) 'Evaluation, Democracy and Social Change', in I. Shaw, J. Greene and M. Mark (eds), *The Sage Handbook of Evaluation*, London: Sage Publications, pp. 118–140

Gretschel, A. (2016) 'Developing the Evaluation of Web-based and Near Services of Youth Work', in A. Gretschel, P. Junttila-Vitikka and A. Puuronen, *Guidelines for Defining and Evaluating the Youth Affairs Sector*, Helsinki: Finnish Youth Research Network/Society, pp. 63–113

House, E. (2005) 'The Many Forms of Democratic Evaluation', in *The Evaluation Exchange*, Vol. XI(3), p. 6; accessed at www.hfrp.org/var/hfrp/storage/original/application/86b58e cfa2fcabb5d74846ffb2edf284.pdf (21.07.16)

House, E. (1980) *Evaluating with Validity*, Thousand Oaks, CA: Sage Publications

House, E., and Howe, K. (1999) *Values in Evaluation and Social Research*, Thousand Oaks, CA: Sage Publications

Howe, K. and Ashcraft, C. (2005) 'Deliberative Democratic Evaluation: Successes and Limitations of an Evaluation of School Choice', *Teachers College Record*, Vol. 107(10), pp. 2274–2297

Johnson, V. (2010) 'Rights Through Evaluation and Understanding Children's Realities', in B. Percy-Smith and N. Thomas (eds), *A Handbook of Children and Young People's Participation*, Abingdon: Routledge, pp. 154–163

Labin, S., Duffy, J., Meyers, D., Wandersman, A. and Lesesne, C. (2012) 'A Research Synthesis of the Evaluation Capacity Building Literature', *American Journal of Evaluation*, Vol. 33(3), pp. 307–338

Love, A. and Muggah, B. (2005) 'Using Democratic Evaluation Principles to Foster Citizen Engagement and Strengthen Neighborhoods', *The Evaluation Exchange*, Vol. XI(3), pp. 14–15 accessed at www.hfrp.org/var/hfrp/storage/original/application/86b58ecfa2f cabb5d74846ffb2edf284.pdf (21.07.16)

MacDonald, B. (1976) 'Evaluation and the Control of Education', in D. Tawney (ed.), *Curriculum Evaluation Today: Trends and Implications*, London: Macmillan Education, pp. 125–136

McTaggart, R. (1991) 'When Democratic Evaluation Doesn't Seem Democratic', *Evaluation Practice*, Vol. 12(1), pp. 9–21

Miller, R. and Campbell, R. (2006), 'Taking Stock of Empowerment Evaluation: An Empirical Review', *American Journal of Evaluation*, Vol. 27(3), pp. 296–319

Orr, S. (2010) 'Exploring Stakeholder Values and Interests in Evaluation', *American Journal of Evaluation*, Vol. 31(4), pp. 557–569

O'Sullivan, R. (2004) *Practicing Evaluation: A Collaborative Approach*, London: Sage Publications

Patton, M. (2005) 'Toward Distinguishing Empowerment Evaluation and Placing It in a Larger Context: Take Two', *American Journal of Evaluation*, Vol. 26(3), pp. 408–414

Reed, M. (2008) 'Stakeholder Participation for Environmental Management: A Literature Review', *Biological Conservation*, Vol. 141(10), pp. 2417–2431

Rodríguez-Campos, L. (2012) 'Advances in Collaborative Evaluation', *Evaluation and Program Planning*, Vol. 35, pp. 523–528

Rodríguez-Campos, L. (2005) *Collaborative Evaluations: A Step-by-Step Model for the Evaluator*, Tamarac, FL: Llumina Press

Rodríguez-Campos, L. and Rincones-Gómez, R. (2013) *Collaborative Evaluations Step-by-Step* (2nd ed.), Stanford, CA: Stanford University Press

Ryan, K. (2005) 'Democratic Evaluation Approaches for Equity and Inclusion', *The Evaluation Exchange*, Vol. XI(3), pp. 2–3 accessed at www.hfrp.org/var/hfrp/storage/original/application/86b58ecfa2fcabb5d74846ffb2edf284.pdf (21.07.16)

Ryan, K. (2004) 'Serving Public Interests in Educational Accountability: Alternative Approaches to Democratic Evaluation', *American Journal of Evaluation*, Vol. 25(4), pp. 443–460

Shulha, L., Whitmore, E., Cousins, J.B., Gilbert, N. and Hudib, H. (2016) 'Introducing Evidence-based Principles to Guide Collaborative Approaches to Evaluation: Results of An Empirical Process, *American Journal of Evaluation*, Vol. 37(2), pp. 193–215

Smith, N. (2007) 'Empowerment Evaluation as Evaluation Ideology', *American Journal of Evaluation*, Vol. 28(2), pp. 169–178

Stufflebeam, D. (1994) 'Empowerment Evaluation, Objectivist Evaluation, and Evaluation Standards: Where the Future of Evaluation Should Not Go and Where It Needs to Go', *Evaluation Practice*, Vol. 15(3), pp. 321–338

Wandersman, A. and Snell-Johns, J. (2005) 'Empowerment Evaluation: Clarity, Dialogue, and Growth', *American Journal of Evaluation*, Vol. 26(3), pp. 421–428

Wandersman, A., Snell-Johns, J., Lentz, B., Fetterman, D., Keener, D., Livet, M., Imm, P. and Flaspohler, P. (2005) 'The Principles of Empowerment Evaluation', in D. Fetterman and A. Wandersman (eds), *Empowerment Evaluation Principles in Practice*, New York: Guilford, pp. 27–41

Weiss, C. (2005) *The Evaluation Exchange*, Vol. XI(3), p. 1

Weiss, C. (1998) 'Have We Learned Anything New About the Use of Evaluation?' *American Journal of Evaluation*, Vol. 19(1), pp. 21–33

Whitmore, E., Guijt, I., Mertens, D., Imm, P., Chinman, M. and Wandersman, A. (2006) 'Embedding Improvements, Lived Experiences and Social Justice in Evaluation Practice', in I. Shaw, J. Greene and M. Mark (eds), *The Sage Handbook of Evaluation*, London: Sage Publications, pp. 340–359

6

TRANSFORMATIVE EVALUATION (TE)

Transformative Evaluation is a participatory methodology developed by the author through research to specifically address the challenges of evaluating youth and community work in England (Cooper 2012b). Transformative Evaluation seeks to increase stakeholder involvement, evaluation use and evaluation capacity. The evaluation methodology follows principles common to participatory evaluation, namely participation, learning, negotiation and flexibility (see Chapter 5). The chapter begins by providing the rationale for developing Transformative Evaluation, describing the youth work practice context at the time of development. This is followed by an examination of the theoretical foundations, namely the transformative paradigm, appreciative inquiry, the most significant change technique and practitioner evaluation. The four-stage model is then presented and explained in depth. The chapter concludes with a discussion of the challenges associated with using Transformative Evaluation.

Rationale

The methodology was developed in 2010 in a third-sector youth organisation in England. At that time, youth work was under threat nationally because of the lack of 'evidence' available to demonstrate its value in an environment of reducing public resources. The challenge facing youth work organisations was how they could articulate this value given that the managerialist climate demanded particular forms of evidence; mostly quantitative data generated using quasi-experimental evaluation approaches. As discussed earlier, youth and community work does not lend itself easily to being measured in this way. Additionally, methods such as random-controlled trials and control groups are neither appropriate nor affordable for small-scale projects.

Many organisations were reshaping their working practices in order to make them more 'measurable', for example, the delivery of workshops in preference to delivering more fluid and flexible open access work. Furthermore, the activity of evaluation had been reformed to reduce the involvement of youth workers, many of whom perceived themselves as 'number crunchers' engaged in a process for the benefit of funders (Ellis and Gregory 2008). This created a sense of alienation among workers (Issit and Spence 2005). In essence, the impetus for the development of Transformative Evaluation was a need to create an evaluation methodology that enabled youth workers to take a more active role in evaluating their effectiveness and the impact of their work. To achieve this, youth workers needed to see a value in evaluation for themselves, the young people they work with and their organisations (Cooper 2012a).

The aim was to design a participatory methodology that could generate evidence of impact *and* redistribute the power inherent in the evaluation process in such a way that practitioners could re-engage with what is an essential aspect of their professional practice. Transformative Evaluation set out to offer more than just a new approach to evaluation; it sought to offer a methodology which promotes interaction and communication between stakeholders as a means of enabling learning for all involved. The ongoing dialogue between youth workers, community members (the young people and stakeholders) and local power-holders (managers and trustees) is key to the process. In Transformative Evaluation, youth workers have a central and active role, they are positioned as the 'evaluators', not simply as data collectors. Additionally, the design was shaped to maximise the 'process use' of evaluation (Patton 2008) with the aim that the 'doing' of evaluation would bring about improvements in youth work practice and outcomes. Essentially, the rationale for developing Transformative Evaluation rests on the premise that by transforming the way we 'think' about evaluation, we can transform the way we 'do' evaluation. If we think differently about our role, about the purpose and about the outcomes of evaluation, we can 'act' differently. We can reclaim evaluation as a process that supports learning, and use that learning to challenge the status quo. The impact of this transformation is multi-layered; seen in improving practice in the moment, seen in the generation of practice knowledge, and in the longer term, through the creation of a culture of evaluation built on collaboration and trust between all stakeholders (see Figure 6.1).

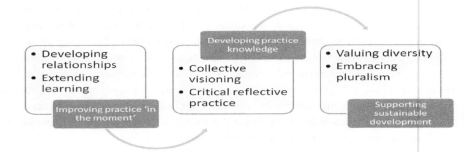

FIGURE 6.1 Transforming evaluation

Theoretical foundations

This Transformative Evaluation model synthesises aspects of the transformative paradigm, appreciative inquiry, most significant change technique and practitioner evaluation. Each aspect is now explored.

The Transformative Paradigm

The underlying philosophical assumptions of the transformative paradigm, summarised in Table 6.1, provided a guide in the design of the Transformative Evaluation methodology.

The central tenet of the transformative paradigm is the inclusion of marginalised groups in evaluation with the aim of achieving social justice. In the context of youth and community work, this not only includes young people and community members but also youth and community workers who have been positioned on the periphery of quasi-experimental evaluation approaches. A commitment to social justice is embedded in Transformative Evaluation. It offers young people and youth and community workers, through their involvement in the generation and analysis of data, a means of influencing local (and potentially, national) decision-makers.

Mertens's (2009) discussion on the use of a deficit perspective in evaluation is important. She warns evaluators to be wary of using deficit models to frame their evaluation design. Deficit models perceive social problems at an individual level rather than a structural or cultural level. In other words, individuals are 'blamed' for social problems, rather than any consideration of how institutional practices or societal responses place certain individuals or groups at increased risk of negative outcomes. This is very pertinent to the context of youth and community work. A belief in the strength of communities is one of the major principles underpinning the Transformative Evaluation paradigm.

Eoyang and Berkas (1999) propose a set of action-orientated principles for guiding Transformative Evaluation design which are summarised below:

- make evaluation a part of the intervention;
- make the evaluation design and processes simple and iterative so they can be easily understood by the stakeholders and involve as many stakeholders as possible in the design;
- make the evaluation processes flexible as they will need to be adapted in situ to take account of the uniqueness of each context; and
- use evaluation as a reinforcing, rather than damping, feedback mechanism.

Two of these principles particularly resonated and offered direction for the development of Transformative Evaluation. Firstly, the idea that the assessment function of evaluation could be part of the intervention – and specifically that this assessment should both enrich and enhance the intervention. If evaluation is experienced as supporting and developing the youth workers' practice with young people, then this is likely to increase their

TABLE 6.1 Philosophical assumptions of the transformative paradigm (from Mertens [2005] cited in Whitmore et al. 2006: 350)

Ontological	Multiple realities shaped by social, political, cultural, ethnic, gender and disability values.
Epistemological	Interactive link between evaluator and stakeholders; knowledge is socially and historically situated; developing a trusting relationship is critical.
Methodological	Inclusion of qualitative (dialogic), but quantitative and mixed methods can be used; contextual and historical factors are described, especially as they relate to oppression.

willingness to actively engage in the process. The second principle that influenced the design of Transformative Evaluation was the use of evaluation to reinforce rather than dampen. This principle encourages the seeking of things to celebrate and to use this to amplify the energy and commitment of those involved. This, again, was very pertinent, given the low morale amongst youth workers at the time.

Evaluation designs informed by the transformative paradigm view evaluation not only as a process that observes change but one that can instigate change (Arvidson and Kara 2013). Some may argue that transformation is an overly ambitious goal for most evaluations; however, Mark (2001) argues that while evaluation may fall short of transformation, it can make a worthwhile contribution towards it.

Appreciative Inquiry (AI)

Appreciative Inquiry (AI) is based on the theoretical framework of positive psychology, and as such it is a strength–based approach. It takes a positive stance in an effort to counterbalance the deficit discourse of problem-solving (Cooperrider and Srivastva 1987; Zandee and Cooperrider 2008). AI has been described as a form of 'constructionism in action' (Reed 2007). Emphasis is placed on language practices on the basis that knowledge construction has more to do with what questions we ask, how we ask them and who is involved, than on what we can 'discover' in terms of matching observation with factual evidence. The fact that we make choices about these things (the 'what', 'who' and 'how') is hightlighted. AI argues that if we ask questions about problems, we create a reality of problems. Alternatively, if we ask questions about what works or what gives life to a community, group, or individual, we participate in the construction of a reality of potential. Mertens (2009) argues that AI is well suited to be applied for transformative purposes because it focuses on the strengths rather than the deficits in a community. Additionally, it offers a process that enhances workers' sense of well-being as it supports:

> the development of action and learning processes based on valuing and building upon what works, what makes us feel good, what we perceive as positive, and what gives us a sense of strength and well-being in the work we do. (Marchi 2011: 181)

AI is guided by five principles:

- the constructivist principle (knowledge is socially constructed);
- the principle of simultaneity (inquiry and change are simultaneous);
- the poetic principle (people author their world);
- the anticipatory principle (the way people shape the future will inform the way they move towards the future); and
- the positive principle (focusing on achievements enables a deeper and longer engagement).

Reed (2007: 27–29) developed a set of presuppositions to support the enactment of these principles, as summarised below:

- in every society, organisation, or group, something works;
- what we focus on becomes our reality;
- reality is created in the moment and there are multiple realities;
- the act of asking questions of an organisation or group influences the group in some way;
- people have more confidence and comfort to journey to the future (the unknown) when they carry forward parts of the past (known);
- if we carry parts of the past forward, they should be what is best about the past;
- it is important to value differences; and
- the language we use creates our reality.

As with any approach, AI has its critics. Some find the positive focus problematic in that 'happy talk' can be used oppressively to prohibit any discussion of difficulties or problems. Reed (2007) responds to this by making clear that AI does not prohibit problem talk, but frames questions that move problem talk towards appreciation and possibilities. Bushe (2007) addresses the challenge that appreciative inquiry is just 'action research with a positive question' arguing that the difference is that AI focuses on generativity rather than problem-solving. Generativity, in the context of appreciative inquiry, involves the creation of new ideas, perceptions, metaphors or images, that are so compelling that they bring about new actions (Bushe 2010). Generativity shifts the way people see the future and opens up new possibilities.

Most Significant Change (MSC)

The Most Significant Change technique is a dialogical, story-based evaluation tool that was developed by Rick Davies in 1996 to address some of the challenges associated with evaluating a complex, participatory, rural development program in Bangladesh. At the time it was seen as a radical departure from the conventional approach of monitoring against prescribed quantitative indicators. It involves the regular collection and participatory interpretation of stories about change. It is important to note that the central aspect of the method is not the stories themselves, but the participatory deliberation and dialogue that the process involves.

Davies and Dart (2005: 8) describe the method as involving:

> The collection of significant change (SC) stories emanating from the field level, and the systematic selection of the most significant of these stories by panels of designated stakeholders or staff. The designated staff and stakeholders are initially involved by 'searching' for project impact. Once changes have been captured, various people sit down together, read the stories aloud and have regular and often in-depth discussions about the value of these reported changes. When the technique is implemented successfully, whole teams of people begin to focus their attention on program impact.

The key purpose of MSC is to facilitate programme improvement although it does also contribute important information and processes to inform the summative evaluation of programmes. The centrality of values is a distinctive aspect of MSC and dynamic values inquiry is critical to the method. The selection of significant change stories requires stakeholders to engage in an ongoing process of deliberation about the value of individual outcomes. This process of values inquiry takes place throughout the organisation and may, in some cases involve funders and policy-makers. Stories about the impact of interventions are a valuable part of MSC. Over time, they penetrate the organisation's collective memory and enable those associated with the programme to gain and retain a more deeply shared understanding of what is being achieved.

At the time of developing Transformative Evaluation, MSC had not been used in evaluations of youth and community work (personal communication with Davies). Its ability to facilitate a dynamic dialogue between stakeholders, and the fact that people enjoy the storytelling process, meant it had much to offer in this context. Critics have argued that the MSC technique does not address the full breadth of impact, nor does it allow for generalisations. In response, it can be argued that it does not set out to do these things. Dart and Davies (2003) clearly state that is not intended to be used as a stand-alone technique but to be used alongside other evaluation methods.

Practitioner evaluation

Practitioner evaluation was first developed by Lawrence Stenhouse (1975) who argues that practitioners are the best judges of their own practice. Practitioner evaluation sits between empowerment evaluation and reflective practice and as such is often associated with an action research methodology (Reason and Bradbury 2000). It shares its foundations with practitioner research which McLeod (1999: 8) defines as 'research carried out by practitioners for the purpose of advancing their own practice. Practitioner evaluation, as a process, supports practitioners to develop knowledge 'in practice' as they reflect on the dynamic interactions between themselves as 'knowers', the beneficiaries of the service as 'knowers', and the established professional knowledge. Moving beyond everyday observation, practitioner evaluation takes the form of a self-reflexive experimental process (Shulman 1997). In essence, it has three elements:

- a commitment to systematic questioning of one's own practice as a basis for development;
- a commitment and the skills to examine one's own practice and the practice of others; and
- a concern to question and to test theory in practice.

Shaw (2011) developed the concept of 'Evaluating in Practice' (EiP) in the field of social work in England. He identified three forms of evaluation:

- external evaluation of practice which is conducted by an external evaluator;
- internal evaluation of practice by practitioners and/or service users; and
- evaluation in practice (EiP).

He describes EiP as what practitioners do when they assess, plan, intervene or review for, and with, service-users. In other words, evaluation is a dimension of everyday practice, not separate from it. EiP can be viewed as an extended and elaborated form of critical reflection, and while it is primarily concerned with strengthening practitioner knowledge and practice, it also supports service-user engagement with practice.

Shaw (2011: 73–74) developed six rules for good EiP, these are summarised as follows:

1. concentrated critical reflection on one's own practice is essential;
2. practitioners must come to 'know what they know', in other words they must seek to elicit the tacit as far as this is possible;
3. practitioners must begin with the knowledge that service-users bring with them;
4. practitioners should exploit the analogy between qualitative methods and direct practice methods to seek a much wider vision of practice-relevance;
5. a requirement of a model of team work; and
6. practitioners must engage with participatory evaluation with service-users.

There is a growing body of evidence about the positive effects on practitioners of engaging in research and enquiry in the field of teaching which transfer to a youth work context. For example, Dadds (1995) and McLaughlin, Black-Hawkins and McIntyre (2004) report that practitioners gain a better understanding of their own practice and ways to improve it, an enhanced understanding of the users' perspective of the service being delivered, and a renewed feeling of pride and excitement about their profession. Additionally, engagement in practitioner evaluation can restore practitioners' sense of professionalism and power in terms of having a voice (McLaughlin et al. 2004).

Transformative Evaluation in practice

Originally Transformative Evaluation was conceived as a four-stage process (see Figure 6.2). The stages are as follows:

- The initial stage involves youth workers and young people generating stories of change. These are termed 'significant change' stories or SC stories.
- In the second stage the youth workers come together as a group to collectively analyse these stories in terms of their content. The youth workers add their commentary to the stories, and these co-authored stories are termed 'contextualised significant change' stories or CSC stories. The youth workers then select a number of the CSC stories to be forwarded to a stakeholder's group for stage three of the process.
- In stage three, the stakeholders analyse the CSC stories received from the youth workers' group. They collectively select one story and provide feedback to the youth workers group explaining the reason for their choice. This story is termed the 'most significant change' story or MSC story.
- Stage four is shown as a process of meta-evaluation. In practice, meta-evaluation takes place as part of each of the previous three stages and thus representing this as a separate stage is perhaps misleading. The rationale for including this

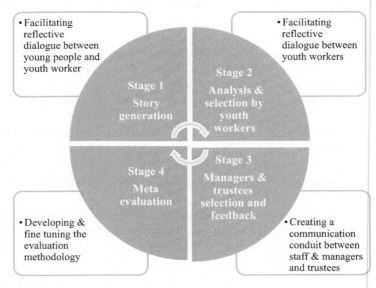

FIGURE 6.2 The Transformative Evaluation model (Cooper 2014)

as a separate stage in the model was to ensure sufficient attention is given to reviewing the process.

It is suggested that one cycle (including the four stages) takes place over a period of three to four months, but this timeframe is flexible and needs to take account of the size of the project being evaluated. The ideal number of youth workers is around five or six as this enables a sufficient number of stories to be generated, and a diversity of views to be expressed during the analysis and selection stage. The stakeholders group may be smaller, in practice, these have tended to include between three and five individuals. The selection of stakeholders is an important consideration as their involvement will lead to a greater understanding of the project's work. Generally, a stakeholder group may include local politicians, commissioners, allied professionals and partners and community representatives.

The process of Transformative Evaluation is reasonably straightforward. However, external facilitation may be needed to support the development of understanding and the skills required for the process to work effectively. External facilitation may be needed to support the development of a culture of critical reflection as this is a crucial aspect of Transformative Evaluation.

The four stages of Transformative Evaluation

Stage 1: Generation of significant change stories

This stage involves youth workers generating significant change stories with the young people they work with. A significant change story is the response to the open question:

> *Looking back, what do you think has been the most significant change that occurred for you as a result of coming here?*

In a single cycle (3–4 months), the aim is for each youth worker to generate four or five stories. This involves facilitating young people to reflect on the outcomes of their involvement with the project, and through these reflective conversations, young people are supported to identify and articulate their learning journey. Importantly, young people's learning is extended or solidified as a result of this process. Generating good quality stories requires good research skills and flexibility. For example, sometimes young people struggle with the word 'significant' because they interpret it in some sort of absolute sense. It can help to ask them to think about what is 'different now' and then to identify what they think is the most significant, in relative terms, of all the changes they have noted.

Significant change stories can be recorded in two ways. Firstly, the youth worker can write notes by hand while they are in conversation with the young person. To strengthen this method, it is essential that the youth worker reads the story back to the young person to check that it reflects their story as they wish to tell it. The story is more valid if it is recorded in the young person's own words. Alternatively, a young person can write their story themselves. Where possible, a story should be written as a simple narrative describing the sequence of events that took place and their significance to the young person.

Generally, young people's stories tend be a paragraph (3 or 4 sentences) but some are much longer and some shorter. The criterion is 'sufficiency', in other words, is there sufficient information contained in the story for the purpose of the evaluation? The story should include the following elements:

- *Description* of the change – What happened? Who did what? When? How?
- *Significance* to the young person of events described in the story. This is a key part of the story. We are interested to know how the young person feels they have changed as a consequence of their engagement, and how this change has come about. Some young people will naturally tell their stories this way, but others may need to be prompted. It is useful to know how this change has impacted on their wider lives beyond the project. This will enable those reading and discussing the story to fully appreciate the significance of the change to the young person.

When generating stories with young people, we must act ethically; we need to be open about what we are doing. It is necessary to explain to young people how their story is to be used and to check that they are happy for their story to be used in that way. Because of the emergent nature of 'narrative', it is good practice to re-confirm consent after the story has been recorded and checked by the young person. Young people should be informed that all the stories are anonymised at stage two and that pseudonyms will be attached to each story. Encouraging the young person to assign the pseudonym themselves supports their understanding of consent and anonymity (see Chapter 8 for a more detailed discussion on ethics).

Stage 2: Youth workers' analysis and selection of contextualised significant change stories

This stage involves three steps: a) identification of domains; b) generating contextualised significant change stories; and c) selection of one contextualised significant change story for each domain.

Step A: Identification of domains

The identification of domains is the first level of analysis. Domains are 'categories of change'; emergent domains are used in Transformative Evaluation (see Chapter 11 for further discussion). Emergent domains are set through a process of sorting the significant change stories into meaningful groups based on their content and then agreeing a title (a domain name) for each group. In other words, the domains

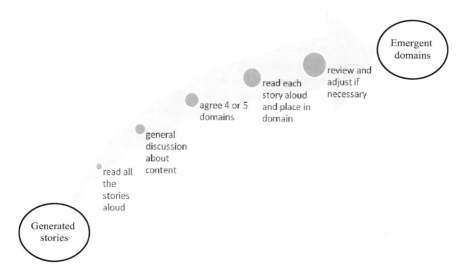

FIGURE 6.3 Creating emergent domains

emerge from the generated stories. The process of determining domains begins with each youth worker reading aloud their generated stories, just as they are written, no ad-libbing or editing, or adding further comment – solely the young people's words. Once all the stores have been read, the group discusses and agrees four or five domain names that generally describe the content of the stories (see Figure 6.3). The stories are read aloud again and each one is placed in the most relevant domain. This discursive process is an important one. It requires sufficient time for the youth workers to listen to and develop understanding of the views of each other in order to reach consensus about the domain names and the positioning of the stories.

It is likely that the number of stories in each domain will be different. This is not a problem; however, should one domain have a large number of stories, for example, more than twelve of the twenty stories on the table, it may be necessary to look again at the domain itself to see whether it is too broad. Conversely, agreeing to too many domains (more than five is probably too many) is also to be avoided. This is sometimes indicative of the group struggling to reach consensus, and if this should happen, the group will need to pay attention to their decision-making process.

Step B: Generating contextualised significant change stories

A contextualised significant change story is created by combining a significant change story with a professional commentary from the youth worker who generated it. In other words, it contains two parts: the young person's narrative and a commentary from the youth worker. The youth worker's commentary adds context to the young person's story, the 'background', and their professional opinion of the significance of the young person's journey of change. The purpose is to provide someone who does not know the young person with as full a picture as possible of the 'distance travelled' and significance of the intervention or interventions that enabled the change. In doing this the youth worker becomes a co-author of the contextualised significant change story.

The workers read aloud the first drafts of their co-authored stories which they prepare in advance of the group meeting and their peers pose questions on the basis of this to facilitate a critical dialogue. This engagement in reflective dialogue supports the co-construction of the story and enables the development of a clear articulation of the young person's outcome and the youth worker's intervention. This process is repeated for each story in the domain and for each domain.

Step C: Selection of one contextualised significant change story for each domain

This step involves the group selection of one contextualised significant change story for each domain. It requires each member of the group to offer their opinion as to which story in a particular domain represents the 'best' example of youth work. They need to explain the reasons for their choice to the group. This requires the full commitment of the group to participate; there should be no opting out or 'social loafing'. Each viewpoint is important and valuable to the group. If it differs it is even more important that it is shared. Through critical discussion, the group identify one story for each domain and a collective reason for their choice is added to the story. This process can feel uncomfortable for some, particularly as those involved in the selection are also those who generated the stories and this will need to be taken account of in the group process.

By the end of stage two of the process, a number of contextualised significant change stories (usually four or five) have been selected. These stories contain the following elements:

- the young person's story in their own words;
- the context and professional commentary added by the youth worker who generated the story; and
- the group's reason for selecting the story as the 'best' example in that domain.

The selected contextualised significant change stories are then presented to the stakeholder group to initiate stage three.

Stage 3: Selection of the most significant change story for the cycle

At this stage, the stakeholder group receive the four or five selected contextualised significant change stories from the youth workers group. Following a similar process used by the youth workers in stage two, the stakeholders read the stories aloud and then engage in critical dialogue as to which story they feel represents the 'best' example of youth work for the cycle. They, too, have to reach consensus through critical discussion. Their collective reason for selection is added to the story they choose. The cycle concludes when the selected story, together with the group's reason for selection, is returned to the youth workers group.

Stage 4: Meta-evaluation

Meta-evaluation is generally understood as the 'evaluation of evaluation'. It often takes the form of an additional external study to authenticate the process or product of an evaluation. Here it is used as a process of informal reviewing during the evaluation (Stake 2004). Reviewing the experience of those involved in the evaluation (the young people, youth workers and stakeholders) can identify any concerns about the methodology that need to be discussed. Additionally, the meta-evaluation stage supports the development of skills and deepens understanding of Transformative Evaluation. Further, this process of ongoing review facilitates an open dialogue and critical discussion about the evaluation findings.

Challenges associated with Transformative Evaluation

Perceived limitations that can be raised in relation to this Transformative Evaluation model are similar to those raised in regards to many other forms of participatory evaluation, namely notions of validity, reliability and generalisability. Criticisms based on these are particularly prevalent at a time when the accountability function is privileged over the other functions of evaluation (learning and improvement). These criticisms are clearly based on positivist-inspired aspirations; TE is informed by the interpretive paradigm and does not draw on these positivist criteria. Instead TE uses interpretive-based criteria such as credibility, transferability, dependability and confirmability to judge evaluation findings (see Chapter 9 for further discussion).

Two concerns may be raised in relation to the use of stories as data; firstly, the use of only positive stories, and secondly, the question as to whether the stories are 'manipulated' by the youth workers' involvement. In response to the first concern, the appreciative underpinning of the methodology is clearly stated from the outset. There are examples of evaluations using the most significant change technique where negative stories were explicitly sought alongside positive stories. However, the decision to take an appreciative approach in Transformative Evaluation was driven by a desire to challenge the deficit discourse of youth and of youth work prevalent in England.

The second concern relating to the process of generating the young people's stories has two aspects; sampling and manipulation. In relation to sampling, TE uses a selective rather than an inclusive process. In other words, it does not seek to provide information on 'average' youth work; it seeks to provide information about particularly successful events. This is referred to as purposive sampling. Purposive sampling may be seen as a weakness in the positivist paradigm; however, the inter-pretivist paradigm views it as a strength. It is entirely appropriate to select 'excellent informants' (Spradley 1979) as these people are the ones who can tell us the most about the question we seek to understand. Selecting young people knowing that they have experienced a change as a result of being involved with the organisation is 'purposefully biased', not to make the organisation look good but in order to learn from those cases of good practice (Patton 2002).

Manipulation is a serious issue that demands attention. It can be argued that the conversation through which a story is generated is not a conversation between equal partners because the youth worker defines and controls the situation (Kvale and Brinkmann 2009). It is they who record, analyse and present the data. At any stage of the process, the young person's voice can be silenced, raised or manipulated. Conversations between young people and youth workers are not power-neutral (Fontana and Frey 2005). As such, it is necessary to consider issues of power, par-ticularly in light of any claim to participation and collaboration. Youth workers need to be sensitive to the power relations that exist in the conversations as these will be embedded in the stories they produce (Briggs 2003).

While the relationships that exist between youth workers and young people can provide privileged access to young people's views, opinions and lived experience, they may also unduly influence what young people say. This raises a question of how can we know they are telling 'their' story rather than what they might think we want to hear? Is there always only one story to tell or do young people have several to choose from? If it is the latter, then what influences their choice? There are no right answers to these thought-provoking questions; this is a matter for professional judgement and awareness. Youth workers need to be able to resist the urge to fall for flattery and instead, continually examine their influence and think about how they can reduce this by using probing questioning techniques.

Tried and tested

Since its inception in 2012, Transformative Evaluation has been used by the author in a number of youth work organisations in the UK, Europe and Australia. In 2016, the methodology was used in an Erasmus-funded project to develop and commu-nicate the impact of youth work in Finland, Estonia, France, Italy and England. Further projects in Scotland and Western Australia began in 2017. Overall, more than a thousand stories of the difference youth work makes to the lives of young people have been generated using this model. TE was originally developed to support organisations and youth workers to engage in evaluation. Its use, however, goes beyond this. Importantly, the stories produced by the process provide a wealth of information, and content analysis of these stories has provided a significant body of evidence to support the value of youth work in a range of contexts and coun-tries. The evidence-base created offers a significant contribution to demonstrating the value of youth and community work to a wide audience. Further, it has the potential to be used to influence policy-makers and funders.

References

Arvidson, M. and Kara, H. (2013) Putting Evaluations to Use: From Measuring to Endorsing Social Value, Working paper 110, London: Third Sector Research Council, accessed at www.birmingham.ac.uk/generic/tsrc/documents/tsrc/working-papers/working-paper-110.pdf (21.07.16)

Briggs, C. (2003) 'Interviewing, Power/Knowledge and Social Inequality', in J. Holstein and J. Gubrium (eds), *Inside Interviewing: New Lenses, New Concerns*, London: Sage Publications, pp. 495–506

Bushe, G. (2010) 'Generativity and the Transformational Potential of Appreciative Inquiry', in D. Zandee, D. Cooperrider and M. Avital (eds), *Organizational Generativity: Advances in Appreciative Inquiry*, Volume 3, Bingley, UK: Emerald Group Publishing Ltd

Bushe, G. (2007) 'Appreciative Inquiry is Not (Just) About the Positive', *OD Practitioner*, Vol. 39(4), pp. 30–35

Cooper, S. (2014) 'Putting Collective Reflective Dialogue at the Heart of the Evaluation Process', in *Reflective Practice*, Vol. 15(5), pp. 563–578

Cooper, S. (2012a) 'Evaluation: Ensuring Accountability or Improving Practice?', in J. Ord (ed.), *Critical Issues in Youth Work Management*, London: Routledge, pp. 82–95

Cooper, S. (2012b) 'Transformative Evaluation: An Interpretive Study of Youth Workers' Experience of Using Participatory Evaluation', Doctoral Thesis, available at https://ore.exeter.ac.uk/repository/handle/10036/3759

Cooperrider, D. and Srivastva, S. (1987) 'Appreciative Inquiry in Organisational Life', in R. Woodman and W. Pasmore (eds), *Research in Organisational Change and Development*, Vol. 1, Stamford, CT: JAI Press, pp. 129–169

Dadds, M. (1995) *Passionate Enquiry and School Development: Story About Teacher Action Research*, Abingdon: Routledge

Dart, J. and Davies, R. (2003) 'A Dialogical, Story-based Evaluation Tool: The Most Significant Change Technique', in *American Journal of Evaluation*, Vol. 24(2), pp. 137–155

Davies, R. and Dart, J. (2005) The 'Most Significant Change' (MSC) technique. A guide to its use, accessed at www.mande.co.uk/docs/MSCGuide.pdf (21.07.16)

Ellis, J. and Gregory, T. (2008) *Accountability and Learning: Developing Monitoring and Evaluation in the Third Sector*, London: Charities Evaluation Services

Eoyang, G. and Berkas, T. (1999) 'Evaluating Performance in a Complex Adaptive System', in M. Lissack, and H. Gunz (eds), *Managing Complexity in Organizations: A View in Many Directions*, Westport, CT: Quorum Books, pp. 313–316

Fontana, A. and Frey, J. (2005) 'The Interview: From Neutral Stance to Political Involvement', in N. Denzin and Y. Lincoln (eds), *The Sage Handbook of Qualitative Research* (3rd ed.), London: Sage Publications, pp. 695–727

Issitt, M. and Spence, J. (2005) 'Practitioner Knowledge and Evidence-based Research, Policy and Practice', in *Youth & Policy*, Vol. 88, pp. 63–82

Kvale, S. and Brinkmann, S. (2009) *Interviews: Learning the Craft of Qualitative Research Interviewing* (2nd ed.), London: Sage Publications

Marchi, S. (2011) 'Co-constructing an Appreciative and Collective Eye: Appreciative Reflection in Action in Lifelong Career Guidance', *Reflective Practice*, Vol. 12(2), pp. 179–194

Mark, M. (2001) 'Evaluation's Future: Furor, Futile, Or Fertile?', *American Journal of Evaluation*, Vol. 22(3), pp. 457–479

McLaughlin, C., Black-Hawkins, K. and McIntyre, D. (2004) Researching Teachers, Researching Schools, Researching Networks: A Summary of the Literature, accessed at www.educ.cam.ac.uk/research/projects/super/ReviewOfLiterature.pdf (25.08.17)

McLeod, J. (1999) *Practitioner Research in Counselling*, London: Sage Publications

Mertens, D. (2009) *Transformative Research and Evaluation*, New York: Guilford Press

Patton, M. (2008) *Utilization-focused Evaluation* (4th ed.), London: Sage Publications

Patton, M. (2002) *Qualitative Research and Evaluation Methods* (3rd ed.), London: Sage Publications

Reason, P. and Bradbury, H. (2000) *Handbook of Action Research: Participatory Inquiry and Practice*, London: Sage Publications

Reed, J. (2007) *Appreciative Inquiry: Research for Change*, London: Sage Publications

Shaw, I. (2011) *Evaluating in Practice*, Farnham: Ashgate Publishing Ltd

Shulman, L.(1997) 'Disciplines of Inquiry in Education: A New Overview', in R. Jaeger (ed.), *Complementary Methods for Research in Education* (2nd ed.), Washington: American Educational Research Association, pp. 3–29

Spradley, J. (1979) *The Ethnographic Interview*, New York: Holt, Rinehart and Winston

Stake, R. (2004) 'Stake and Responsive Evaluation', in C. Alkin (ed.), *Evaluation Roots, Tracing Theorists' Views and Influences*, Thousand Oaks, CA: Sage Publications

Stenhouse, L. (1975) *An Introduction to Curriculum Development and Research*, London: Heinemann

Whitmore, E., Guijt, I., Mertens, D., Imm, P., Chinman, M. and Wandersman, A. (2006) 'Embedding Improvements, Lived Experiences and Social Justice in Evaluation Practice', in I. Shaw, J. Greene and M. Mark (eds), *The Sage Handbook of Evaluation*, London: Sage Publications, pp. 340–359

Zandee, D., and Cooperrider, D. (2008) 'Appreciable Worlds, Inspired Inquiry', in P. Reason and H. Bradbury (eds), *Handbook of Action Research* (2nd ed.), London: Sage Publications, pp. 190–198

7

LEARNING IN PARTICIPATORY EVALUATION

Introduction

The focus of the concluding chapter of this part of the book is on learning. Learning is one of the three functions of evaluation; the other two are accountability and project development. It has been argued that the dominant discourse of evaluation since the mid-1990s has been one of accountability, and that this has led to the relegation of the learning function of evaluation (see Chapter 1 and 2). There has been much discussion about if, and how, these three functions can co-exist within evaluation and this chapter begins with a discussion of the contentions. The focus of this chapter is on learning, and in particular, the learning that arises from the engagement in evaluation as opposed to learning that is gained from the results of evaluation. Three examples from practice are used to illustrate the potential for this form of learning in participatory evaluation.

Learning and accountability: a dichotomy?

As noted in Chapter 1, evaluation has three functions:

- an accountability function that seeks to respond to the question of whether contractual agreements have been met;
- a programme development function which focuses on improving the quality of the programme;
- a learning function that aims to develop understanding about what forms of practice are successful. (Chelminsky 1997)

Discussions on whether evaluation should privilege learning over accountability or accountability over learning, is a source of controversy (Picciotto 2016). There are those who feel that the accountability and learning functions are irreconcilable. Evaluations can only focus on one or the other. Arguably this depends on how accountability is conceptualised. For example, when evaluation is experienced as a tool for 'blaming and shaming' or when it is experienced as a threat, then clearly it will bring about a defensive response rather than an openness to learning. However, if accountability is perceived more broadly, if it is seen less as upward compliance and more about being accountable to all stakeholders and self, then accountability and learning may sit more comfortably together. Heider (2016a) questions whether 'accountability' and 'learning' have become the next big dichotomy for evaluation, replacing the quantitative/qualitative arguments of the past. She suggests that instead of focusing on separating the learning and accountability functions of evaluation, attention is given to the deeper issues that stand in the way of learning. She argues that 'Corporate culture or attitudes towards and of evaluation play an important part in shaping how evaluation can be effective in influencing change with a balance of learning and accountability' (Heider 2016b: 14). These debates will, no doubt, continue for some time yet. They may be a 'distraction', diverting our attention away from the deeper issues as Heider suggests, however, they may also promote a dialogue through which a deeper understanding of the learning potential of evaluation can emerge.

Learning in evaluation

All forms of evaluation can be viewed as systematic ways of learning from experience, indeed 'evaluation makes little sense unless it is understood as part of a learning process' (Rowe and Taylor 2005: 205). However, as Patton (2008) points out, learning from evaluation is often taken to mean learning from the results of evaluation. He argues that learning from engaging in evaluation itself (what he calls 'process use') is distinct from learning that arises from findings presented in evaluation reports. The chapter begins by exploring 'process use' and examines the different forms this can take. These ideas are then expanded by using examples from practice to illustrate the value of 'process use' in youth and community work.

Learning from engaging in evaluation is clearly different to learning from reading an evaluation report; both are valid and valuable forms of learning. Patton (2008) uses the term 'process use' to describe the learning gained from engaging in evaluation, and to distinguish it from the learning gained from the results or products of evaluation. Patton (2008: 155) describes 'process use' learning as: 'the individual changes in thinking, attitudes and behaviours, (...) that occur among those individuals involved in evaluation as a result of the learning that occurs during the evaluation process.'

It is in the process of the evaluation that this learning occurs and as such, participatory forms of evaluation are ideally suited to offer opportunities for learning. The focus on process, dialogue and reflection arguably provide enhanced learning opportunities for all involved. Process use can occur at organisation level, for example, the process of stakeholders socially constructing their reality through participatory evaluation enhances organisational learning significantly (Cousins and Earl 1992). Suárez-Herrera, Springett and Kagan (2009) go further, suggesting that the interaction and communication between stakeholders engaged in evaluative networks constitute a superior way of learning.

Five types of 'process use'

Building on Patton's earlier work, Forrs, Rebien and Carlsson (2002) developed a typology of five types of learning that can arise from engaging in evaluation, rather than from evaluation findings or reports. These are:

1. learning to learn;
2. developing professional networks;
3. creating shared understandings;
4. strengthening the project; and
5. boosting morale.

Each is now explored in relation to participatory evaluation in youth and community work.

Learning to learn

'Learning to learn' is generally understood as a process of discovery about learning. It is through this process of discovery that people develop both the skills and, more importantly, the disposition, to support learning across their lifespan. Learning to learn has become a popular concept in the twenty-first century as a consequence of the rapid pace of change. In this context, knowledge itself is not what we need, instead we need the ability to continually learn. There are a number of linked capabilities, for example, curiosity, criticality and reflection (Claxton 2007).

In participatory evaluation, learning to learn relates to developing evaluative skills and the readiness and willingness (disposition) to put those skills to work. For youth and community workers, the 'learning to learn' process is closely aligned with the concept of reflective practice; both require curiosity, criticality and reflection. Participatory evaluation approaches can provide a welcome space for reflection at a time when managerialism has eroded reflective learning opportunities (Baldwin 2004; Ottesen 2007). Time constraints are also a recognised barrier to reflective practice (Fade 2004; Morris and Stew 2007; Thompson and Thompson 2008). When workloads are high, reflective practice can be seen as a luxury, yet, according to Thompson and Pascal (2012: 320) 'the busier we are, the more reflective we need to be'. Thus, the argument can be made that using participatory evaluation provides practitioners with space, time and 'learn to learn' opportunities that have been lost.

Participatory approaches to evaluation can also provide young people with opportunities for 'learning to learn' by supporting them to reflect on how they have changed and developed over time. The process of engaging in evaluation supports young people to develop skills in reflection. This aligns with Estrella's (2000) proposition that participatory evaluation can be used as a self-assessment tool because it enables people to reflect on past experiences, examine current realities, revisit objectives and define future strategies. Supporting young people to develop their ability to reflect has the potential to enable them to gain a range of associated skills including analytical skills, self-awareness skills, critical thinking skills and communication skills (Thompson and Thompson 2008; Claxton 2007). Being able to see the benefits for young people is likely to be an incentive for youth workers to engage meaningfully with evaluation.

Developing professional networks

Participatory forms of evaluation bring people together and hence provide opportunities to build networks (Forrs et al. 2002). The nature and format of these networks will differ depending on the evaluation type and the range of stakeholders involved. For example, they may involve individuals from different professional groups or they may involve practitioners from different settings within a single organisation. The space for youth and community workers to 'come together' has all but disappeared, and when it does happen the focus is more often than not on leadership-driven agendas and the monitoring of performance against targets. The collaborative space provided by participatory evaluation processes offer youth workers access to valuable learning opportunities that have been lost over time.

Importantly, participatory approaches offer more than the ability to support the development of professional networks – the scope is more expansive than this. Participatory evaluations often bring together a wide range of stakeholders, for example, young people, community members, youth workers and managers. These people rarely meet and often hold stereotypical views of each other. Through participating in the process, people are exposed to the views and opinions of others and as a consequence, develop a greater understanding of difference and of respecting difference. Potentially, these networks (as well as professional networks) nurture expansive patterns of thinking that promote generative learning, which Senge (2006: 14) defines as 'learning that enhances our capacity to create'. Collaboration is a key feature of organisational learning, and Senge (2006: 3) highlights the value in 'learning how to learn together'. However, it must be acknowledged that this social relations aspect adds complexity to the evaluation process and effective management of this is crucial to success (Foreman–Peck and Travers 2015; Patton 2008).

Creating shared understanding

Clearly, differences will exist between the views of stakeholders, for example, between policy makers, commissioners, providers and service-users in regards to notions of value, quality and desired outcomes (Watty 2003; Beresford and Branfield 2006). These differences arise because conceptions of quality are based on personal and social constructs that are informed by our values and our beliefs as to the ultimate purpose of youth and community work. These differences will always exist and are likely to create a degree of tension between stakeholders. They can become exclusionary when one conception is seen as dominant (Ellis and Gregory 2008; Issitt and Spence 2005).

The collaborative nature of participatory evaluation approaches provides a space and structure to explore these tensions. Through collective dialogues, the opportunity to work towards a shared understanding of the nature and purpose of the service being delivered and the most appropriate means of evaluating it, can be realised. Recognition of the value of each stakeholder's perspective is a foundational aspect of creating a shared understanding. Also, engaging in collaborative action enables people to understand the motives of others and to respect differences.

Strengthening the project

Evaluation is all too often conceptualised as a process of looking back, of assessing past performance. However, when a focus is given to learning that can be achieved during the process of the evaluation, this can result in 'real-time' changes, improving practice in the present as well as in the future. For example, in Transformative Evaluation, the engagement of youth and community workers and young people as 'evaluators' embeds the evaluation process in every-day practice in such a way as the process of evaluation enhances learning for both parties. Rather than waiting for the publication of an evaluation report, new understandings may develop that can be acted upon immediately. In other words, the act of evaluating itself can result in improving the quality of practice and the outcomes of practice 'in the moment'. Patton (2008) uses the term 'intervention-orientated evaluation' to describe this integral connection between the generation of evaluation data and the programme outcomes. He argues that evaluation can be seen as an intervention when it supports and reinforces the project's goals and outcomes.

Boosting morale

Boosting morale is not often associated with evaluation. Indeed, youth and community workers, as with many other professionals, have experienced the exact opposite (see Chapter 3). When evaluation is seen as a threat, as something that is imposed and of which they have little control, it can be experienced as undermining. Participatory forms of evaluation offer a different experience. Engaging in collaborative action can generate enthusiasm and commitment and serve to boost morale. The shared ownership of the evaluation process that arises from active participation can restore a sense of professionalism. It can provide youth and community workers with a space for their 'professional voice' and generate a feeling of being valued. When evaluation is conceptualised as something that 'belongs to us' rather than something that is 'imposed on us' by others, there is a shift in the balance of power. The empowering nature of participatory evaluation enables youth and community workers to be active agents in shaping their professional practice and professional contexts (Cooper 2014).

In summary, process use (learning from engaging in evaluation) is aligned with a constructionist learning paradigm as it focuses on the ways in which people make meanings *during* the evaluation. Through dialogue and reflection that promotes a questioning of assumptions, values and beliefs, individuals develop a deeper understanding of the project, the practice, themselves, each other and of evaluation.

Examples from practice

As in Chapter 3, this section of the chapter draws on the doctoral research conducted with youth and community workers in England (Cooper 2012). To recap, in the research, six youth and community workers were interviewed prior to using a participatory evaluation approach and again, twelve months later. During the interim period, they implemented three cycles of Transformative Evaluation. Transformative Evaluation (TE) is a participatory evaluation approach to generate evidence of impact. It involves young people, youth and community workers and stakeholders in the generation of co-constructed stories of change. This approach is explored in depth in Chapter 6. Here, data from the second set of interviews are used to explore three outcomes resulting from their engagement in the evaluation:

- learning in the moment;
- collective reflective practice; and
- empowerment.

Direct quotations from the interview transcripts are used and these are shown in italics.

Learning in the moment

Two examples are presented to illustrate the potential of immediate impact on practice occurring as a consequence of 'doing' evaluation, rather than as a result of the analysis of evaluation findings. The first of these examples draws on the workers' experience of the story generation stage of the methodology (see Chapter 6 for more detail on the methodology). The youth and community workers were interviewed after using Transformative Evaluation for twelve months. In that time, they had completed three cycles of the methodology and generated, on average, fifteen stories each.

The workers reported that the process of generating stories had enhanced their existing relationships with young people and thus improved practice 'in the moment'. Generating significant change stories involved the youth workers facilitating young people to reflect on the outcome of their involvement with the project, illuminating their learning journeys. This reflective process enabled workers to develop deeper relationships with young people, as one youth worker stated:

> *Because you're asking them questions which are kind of difficult, rather than just offhand comments about things, you create a bit more of a relationship, you develop your relationship with people a bit more.*

Another worker reflected:

> *The stories they told were meaningful to both of us, from the experiences that had gone on in the Centre, so there was a bit of bonding there whilst we discussed the stories.*

Importantly, learning for the young person and the youth and community worker is possibly extended or solidified as a result of the evaluation process. This was expressed very well when one worker said '*the process of generating the story is a journey in itself*'.

The second example relates to the youth workers' 'theories of action' (Argyris and Schön 1974). It demonstrates how the evaluation process identified the gap between the workers' espoused theory and their theory-in-use. The espoused theory of youth and community work is that conversation and dialogue is central to our practice as informal educators (Jeffs and Smith 2005; Batsleer 2008). It is through dialogue that we create opportunities for learning; conversations *are* our interventions. The TE methodology was developed on this premise, the assumption being that youth workers could generate significant change stories through these conversations with young people. However, surprisingly, many of the workers commented on how much they had enjoyed the experience of 'sitting down and talking' with young people. This was unexpected, particularly as the espoused theory is that 'sitting down and talking' with young people is an everyday activity for youth workers. This, however, did not seem to be the case, as one worker's comment illustrates:

> *you knew you had to do it* [generate stories] *and I think if we didn't have to do it, it* [the conversation] *wouldn't have happened.*

The process of evaluation illuminated the theory-in-use. The workers talked about the difficulty in finding time to engage in meaningful conversation with young people. In some cases, they expressed a reluctance to engage in deeper conversations with young people on the basis that these conversations would likely be interrupted by their need to deal with other things, most notably behaviour management. This raised important questions for the youth workers involved, their organisation and the wider youth work field. If meaningful conversation is central to youth work, and yet workers were not engaging in this activity, what are the reasons for this, what is happening instead? What does this mean for youth work? Illuminating the gap between the espoused theory and the theory-in-use prompted change, as illustrated by the reflective comments made by one youth worker:

One thing I will take away from this is to make sure we give the opportunity to young people and that we take the opportunity ourselves to be able to sit down and talk to them about either why they come or how they feel they progress, how they feel they're getting on, it's definitely made me want to take more time to do that.

In summary, the learning gained from their engagement in the process of evaluation enhanced the youth workers' practice 'in the moment'. It enabled them to spend quality time with young people, in meaningful conversations, that developed and deepened their relationships with young people. It required them to prioritise time to engage in one-to-one reflective conversations with young people and validated the activity of 'sitting down and talking'. The evaluation promoted the process of 'really talking' (Belenky 1986 cited in Mezirow 2000: 14) and 'generous listening' (Reed 2007: ix). Emphasis is placed on active listening, reciprocity and co-operation, and active dialogue is used to better understand the meaning and value of an experience. Further, the evaluation provided a frame to support the development of meaningful conversations; a template that aided a shift from everyday surface conversation to deeper and more meaningful educative conversations that constitute skilful youth work.

Learning through collective reflection

The youth workers using the Transformative Evaluation methodology found the process re-united them with reflective practice. It highlighted the fact that their engagement with reflective practice had decreased. For example, one worker explained:

sometimes you just slog on and don't really think about what you're doing, or all the stuff you've done (...) that kind of gets forgotten.

Another worker talked about a need to make more time to reflect on his practice, and for him, this included talking with young people about what they had done and what they had achieved. These workers are expressing their learning in terms of 'disposition' rather than skill enhancement, in that their learning has resulted in a greater inclination towards reflective practice.

The act of engaging young people in reflective conversations enabled the youth workers to identify their own assumptions about the outcomes of their work. These reflective conversations enable them to *'find out stuff they didn't know before'* and through this to highlight the differences between what they had assumed young people had taken from a particular intervention and the young person's account of it as shown by the following quotation from a youth worker reflecting on her experience of using TE:

Just reminiscing [with the young person] *about that experience, for both of us was really interesting, and her perspective of that experience was different to what mine was, we had a different view of the outcome.*

As Allard, Goldblatt, Kemball, Kendrick, Millen and Smith (2007) assert, the use of narratives can be a useful vehicle for uncovering assumptions and embedding this in the evaluation process may restore or revitalise the youth workers' desire to reflect with young people, and to recognise the dangers of assumptions that can lead to normative practice.

The collective nature of the methodology was appreciated by the youth and community workers. For example, one worker placed high value on stage two of the process in which they were able to intuitively question each other, negotiate and create shared meanings. She described this as a supervision-type process rather than an evaluation process, indicating its reflective, educative and supportive nature. Another worker elaborated on the in-depth discussions that took place in this peer space as follows:

> ... discussing why a story should go through and why it shouldn't and finding out what everyone thought, either individually or as a group as to what is distance travelled and what is an achievement for a young person and working out who has come the furthest and who has achieved the most.

In the context of youth and community work, concepts such as 'distanced travelled' and young people's achievements are complex. The comments above illustrate a key characteristic of critical reflective learning in that they evidence the move away from the immediate to take a broader view of practice. This shift can be seen to represent a move from adaptive learning to generative learning (Senge 2006), from single-loop to double-loop learning (Argyris and Schön 1978) as the focus of dialogue moves from problem-solving towards active collective reflection on the educational goals, values and issues of equity and social justice (Ng and Tan 2009).

Empowerment

In response to a question relating to the benefits of implementing the evaluation methodology, all the youth workers commented on how it had encouraged and supported them and confirmed their sense of professional self. Woven through the youth workers' accounts were indications of emerging confidence and a belief in the possibility of a level of professional autonomy. One worker expressed his feelings thus:

> The fact is you've got something there that you can actually look at and say 'wow, we've made a difference' so it actually reinforces your work, makes the workforce a lot happier, we're doing the right thing and it gives us confidence in what we're doing.

Another youth worker talked about how her engagement in the process of evaluation had enabled her to recognise the value of her work:

> A bit of a pat on the back because of the things that are happening for young people (...) it's the time we've spent talking about it, time spent reflecting and making ourselves realise that the work we're doing is really important.

An increased sense of self-belief can help support professionals to use their agency (Osgood 2006) and one worker demonstrated her sense of increased agency when she said:

> *It will give us ammunition to justify the work that we do, when you're told from above that you can't do something anymore, you'll be able to turn around and say it might not be hitting those targets but this is what it's generating.*

This sense of improved well-being and agency is associated with the appreciative underpinning of the Transformative Evaluation methodology. The 'appreciative gaze' (Ghaye, Melander-Wikman, Kisare, Chambers, Bergmark, Kostenius, and Lillyman 2008; Reed 2007) turned the focus to the things that worked and countered the effects of performativity. Rather than focusing on the problems and the associated feeling of inadequacy, the workers were able to see the positive nature of their work and feel good about that, leading to an enhanced sense of professional self. At a time when youth and community work is going through radical change, and when professionalism and professional identity is under threat, a process that enables practitioners to feel positive about themselves and about the work they do, must have advantages for young people, practitioners and the organisation overall.

The morale boosting aspect, one of the five types of learning that arises from engagement in evaluation, can be seen in the extracts below:

> *It has made me feel that actually there was some really good stories that came out of there and you know, even when it's really crappy, for young people it is valuable for them.*
>
> *Finding that actually it's really lovely to spend some time doing this, it feels good and I leave the meetings elated and feeling stress-free instead of leaving the meetings feeling 'arrgh, I've got loads to do', it is helping us as individuals.*

These extracts provide support for the view that participatory forms of evaluation can result in a renewed feeling of pride and excitement about the profession and in a revitalised sense of oneself as a professional (Dadds 1995; McLaughlin, Black-Hawkins and McIntyre 2004).

In summary, the focus of this chapter has been on communicating the learning potential of 'doing' evaluation, and as such, it has examined the learning for those actively engaged in the process of evaluation. Importantly, participatory approaches to evaluation offer learning opportunities to all those involved; the young people, youth workers and stakeholders.

Learning at the micro level (between young people and youth and community workers) and at the mezzo (project) level has been described through the use of practice examples. When participatory evaluations include a wider range of participants, for example, commissioners and policy-makers then the process use of evaluation (learning through engaging) can potentially extend to the macro level.

The Deliberative Day Discussion approach used to evaluate youth work provision in Finland provides a good example of this (see Chapter 5). Macro level learning also relates to the learning for others beyond the project or locality. This tends to arises from the 'product' rather than the 'process' of evaluation and thus, has not been explored in this chapter. Generally, macro level learning is achieved via the evaluation report, its dissemination as well as the generation of a body of evidence from multiple evaluations (see Chapter 12).

It is important to understand that learning can occur not only through the 'product' of evaluation but also through the 'process' of evaluation. For those looking to promote the use of participatory approaches to evaluation, the learning potential of 'engaging in the evaluation' provides a strong rationale. In the context of evaluating youth and community work, the concepts of 'process' and 'product' are generally well understood. Youth and community workers are well-positioned to identify the 'process use' of participatory evaluation and to use this to support an argument for its increased use.

References

Allard, C., Goldblatt, P., Kemball, J., Kendrick, S., Millen, J. and Smith, D. (2007) 'Becoming a Reflective Community of Practice', *Reflective Practice*, Vol. 8(3), pp. 299–314

Argyris, C. and Schön, D. (1978) *Organizational Learning: A Theory of Action Perspective*, Reading, MA: Addison Wesley

Argyris, C. and Schön, D. (1974) *Theory in Practice: Increasing Professional Effectiveness*, San Francisco, CA: Jossey-Bass

Baldwin, M. (2004) 'Critical Reflection: Opportunities and Threats to Professional Learning and Service Development in Social Work Organizations', in N. Gould, and M. Baldwin (eds), *Social Work, Critical Reflection and the Learning Organization*, Aldershot: Ashgate Publishing Ltd, pp. 41–56

Batsleer, J. (2008) *Informal Learning in Youth Work*, London: Sage Publications

Beresford, P. and Branfield, F. (2006) 'Developing Inclusive Partnerships: User-defined Outcomes, Networking and Knowledge – A Case Study', *Health and Social Care in the Community*, Vol. 14(5), pp. 436–444

Chelminsky, E. (1997) 'Thoughts for a New Evaluation Society', in *Evaluation*, Vol. 3(1), pp. 97–118

Claxton, G. (2007) 'Expanding young people's capacity to learn', *British Journal of Educational Studies*, Vol. 55(2), pp. 115–134

Cooper, S. (2014) 'Putting Collective Reflective Dialogue at the Heart of the Evaluation Process', in *Reflective Practice*, Vol. 15(5), pp. 563–578

Cooper, S. (2012) *Transformative Evaluation: An Interpretive Study of Youth Workers' Experience of Using Participatory Evaluation*, Doctoral Thesis, available at https://ore.exeter.ac.uk/repository/handle/10036/3759

Cousins, B., and Earl, L. (1992) 'The Case for Participatory Evaluation', *Educational Evaluation and Policy Analysis*, Vol. 14(4), pp. 397–418

Dadds, M. (1995) *Passionate Enquiry and School Development: Story About Teacher Action Research*, Abingdon: Routledge

Ellis, J. and Gregory, T. (2008) *Accountability and Learning: Developing Monitoring and Evaluation in the Third Sector*, London: Charities Evaluation Services

Estrella, M. (2000) 'Learning from Change', in M. Estrella with J. Bluaret, D. Campilan, J. Gaventa, J. Gonsalves, I. Guijt, D. Johnson and R. Ricafort (eds), *Learning From Change: Issues and Experiences in Participatory Monitoring and Evaluation*, London: Intermediate Technology Publications Ltd, pp. 1–13

Fade, S. (2004) 'Using Interpretative Phenomenological Analysis for Public Health Nutrition and Dietetic Research: A Practical Guide', *Proceedings of the Nutrition Society*, Vol. 63, pp. 647–653

Foreman-Peck, L. and Travers, K. (2015) 'Developing Expertise in Managing Dialogue in the "Third Space": Lessons from a Responsive Participatory Evaluation', *Evaluation*, Vol. 21(3), pp. 344–358

Forss, K., Rebien, C. and Carlsson, J. (2002) 'Process Use of Evaluations: Types of Use that Precede Lessons Learned and Feedback', *Evaluation*, Vol. 8(1), pp. 29–45

Ghaye, T., Melander-Wikman, A., Kisare, M., Chambers, P., Bergmark, U., Kostenius, C. and Lillyman, S. (2008) 'Participatory and Appreciative Action and Reflection (PAAR) – Democratizing Reflective Practices', *Reflective Practice*, Vol. 9(4), pp. 361–397

Heider, C. (2016a) 'Facing Off: Accountability and Learning – the Next Big Dichotomy in Evaluation?', blog at http://ieg.worldbank.org/blog/facing-accountability-and-learning-next-big-dichotomy-evaluation (Tuesday, March 22, 2016 – 10:27)

Heider, C. (2016b) 'Forum: Is There a Trade-off between Accountability and Learning in Evaluation?' in *Evaluation Connections,* European Evaluation Society Newsletter February 2016

Issitt, M. and Spence, J. (2005) 'Practitioner Knowledge and Evidence-based Research, Policy and Practice', *Youth & Policy*, Vol. 88, pp. 63–82

Jeffs, T. and Smith, M. (2005) *Informal Education: Conversation, Democracy and Learning*, Nottingham: Educational Heretics Press

McLaughlin, C., Black-Hawkins, K. and McIntyre, D. (2004) *Researching Teachers, Researching Schools, Researching Networks: A Summary of the Literature*, accessed at www.educ.cam.ac.uk/research/projects/super/ReviewOfLiterature.pdf (25.08.17)

Mezirow, J. (2000) *Learning as Transformation: Critical Perspectives on a Theory in Progress*, San Francisco: Jossey-Bass

Morris, J. and Stew, G. (2007) 'Collaborative Reflection: How Far Do 2:1 Models of Learning in the Practice Setting Promote Peer Reflection?', *Reflective Practice*, Vol. 8(3), pp. 419–432

Ng, P.T. and Tan, C. (2009) 'Communities of Practice for Teachers: Sensemaking or Critical Reflective Learning?', *Reflective Practice*, Vol. 10(1), pp. 37–44

Osgood, J. (2006) 'Professionalism and Performativity: The Feminist Challenge Facing Early Years Practitioners', *Early Years*, Vol. 26(2), pp. 187–199

Ottesen, E. (2007) 'Reflection in Teacher Education', *Reflective Practice*, Vol. 8(1), pp. 31–46

Patton, M. (2008) *Utilization-focused Evaluation* (4th ed.), London: Sage Publications

Picciotto, R. (2016) 'Evaluation is on the Move: An editorial', in *Evaluation Connections,* European Evaluation Society Newsletter February 2016

Reed, J. (2007) *Appreciative Inquiry: Research for Change*, London: Sage Publications

Rowe, M. and Taylor, M. (2005) 'Community-led Regeneration: Learning Loops or Reinvented Wheels?', in D. Taylor and S. Balloch (eds), *The Politics of Evaluation*, Bristol: The Policy Press, pp. 205–222

Senge, P. (2006) *The Fifth Discipline: The Art and Practice of the Learning Organization*, (2nd ed.), London: Random House Business Books

Suárez-Herrera, J., Springett, J. and Kagan, C. (2009) 'Critical Connections between Participatory Evaluation, Organizational Learning and Intentional Change in Pluralistic Organizations', *Evaluation*, Vol. 15(3), pp. 321–342

Thompson, N. and Pascal, J. (2012) 'Developing Critically Reflective Practice', *Reflective Practice*, Vol. 13(2), pp. 311–325

Thompson, S. and Thompson, N. (2008) *The Critically Reflective Practitioner*, Basingstoke: Palgrave Macmillan

Watty, K. (2003) 'When Will Academics Learn about Quality?', *Quality in Higher Education*, Vol. 9(3), pp. 213–221

PART 3

Participatory evaluation in practice

This part of the book focuses on implementing a participatory evaluation approach and seeks to offer guidance to those new to participatory evaluation in youth and community work and a helpful check for those already using a participatory approach.

Chapter 8 ('Preparing for evaluation') takes the reader through the various preparation and planning stages required for an effective evaluation. This begins with clarifying and articulating purpose, leading to the development of a theory of change. Ethical considerations need to be embedded in the evaluation process, and this starts in the planning stage. Planning in relation to identification, recruitment and engagement of stakeholders is discussed and the chapter concludes with a consideration of resources.

Chapter 9 ('Data in participatory evaluation') explores the 'what' and 'how' of data generation in participatory evaluation. It includes a discussion on trustworthiness in the context of participatory evaluation and concludes with a consideration of factors that influence the choice of data generation methods.

Chapter 10 ('Methods for generating data') examines four data generation methods that are often associated with participatory evaluation. These include questionnaires, interviews, observations and story-telling. Each method is critically examined in regards to the type of data that may be generated and in relation to their associated advantages and disadvantages.

Chapter 11 ('Analysing data') seeks to enable youth and community workers to develop their skills and confidence in making use of data. The chapter examines various ways in which generated data can be analysed, with particular emphasis on analysing qualitative data as participatory evaluations tend to generate more qualitative than quantitative data. Content analysis is explained and an example from a Transformative Evaluation is included to illustrate its use.

Chapter 12 ('Sharing knowledge') is the final chapter in this part of the book. It begins with a focus on voice, audience and message. A discussion on report writing follows before moving on to explore more participatory ways of sharing knowledge. The chapter concludes with a section on meta-evaluation to promote an ongoing review of the process in order to develop new understandings of 'what works well' in participatory evaluation.

8

PREPARING FOR EVALUATION

Introduction

While it is true that evaluation can be seen as something we do as a matter of course in our everyday lives, effective evaluation in professional practice requires preparation and planning. This is even more important when a participatory approach to evaluation is used as it involves a number of different people who are likely to have differing perspectives and experiences of the project being evaluated. These perspectives need to be acknowledged and valued for what they bring to the evaluation, yet the evaluation findings need to be presented as a coherent whole. This is no mean feat and time spent during the preparatory stage will pay dividends in the long run.

The preparation stages are outlined in this chapter. It begins with the need to clarify the purpose of the evaluation at the outset. Attending to questions such as 'what is the evaluation for?' and 'what do we want to achieve through the evaluation?' will support the development of a shared understanding of the purpose of the evaluation and provide a framework for the evaluation activities. The focus can then be directed to the project itself, and a theory of change approach can be used to identify the project's aims, processes and outcomes to be evaluated and the most appropriate methods for generating evidence. It is necessary to consider the question of ethics at this early stage. Ethical practice needs to be embedded in the process of evaluation and considered throughout, particularly as participatory evaluation is a dynamic process. It is highly likely that issues will emerge that may not have been foreseen because of the organic nature of participatory evaluation.

The identification, recruitment and engagement of stakeholders is key to participatory evaluation. These actions are rarely straightforward, and they often require a great deal of preparation. Decisions concerning who should be involved, and how, and the roles and responsibilities of the different stakeholder groups will need to be considered and agreed. Attention should also be given to the ways in which these groups will interact with each other. This will involve a consideration of issues of power, potential conflicts and conflict resolution strategies during the planning stage. The chapter concludes with a review of the resourcing requirements of participatory evaluation.

Clarifying and articulating purpose

Being clear about the purpose of the evaluation is essential if you are to engage others in the process. For many, the notion of evaluation is something that is 'done to them' by those in positions of power, often as a requirement of funding agencies. It is likely that stakeholders will assume that the 'evaluator' holds an authoritative role. Thus, there is a need to clearly articulate how participatory evaluation is different. The difference between participatory evaluation and quasi-experimental evaluation should be explained using language that can be understood by all. This will prepare those involved to see evaluation as a collective learning process that aims to be useful to the programme's beneficiaries (young people and their communities), as well as funders, programme managers and staff.

Articulating the value of participatory evaluation to each group of stakeholders is key to engagement. For example, when managers and staff see it as an integral part of project development they are more likely to recognise the benefits of their involvement. Evaluation becomes a process of learning through experience and a process of measuring 'distance travelled' rather than an inspection or a test. For beneficiaries, participatory evaluation takes account of their lived experiences, acknowledging what is important to them rather than a process which starts with assessment criteria generated by those in positions of power, who claim to know what is best. The objectives of the evaluation are set collectively through dialogue at the preparation and planning stage, and should aim to satisfy the needs of all stakeholders. This includes those who are providing the funding, those who receive the funding, those directly responsible for running the programme, and the 'beneficiaries' of the programme. Clarifying and articulating purpose of the evaluation requires skilful facilitation if it is to create an environment for shared interactive learning. Arguably, it is the attitude and values projected by the facilitator that transforms the evaluation from just another exercise in finding out whether the project works or not, to an empowering experience for all concerned (Crishna 2006).

Developing a 'theory of change'

It is not essential to develop a 'theory of change' but for those considering taking a participatory approach to evaluation it does have significant benefits. In Chapter 1, the concept of theory of change was examined. To recap, theory of change (ToC) describes a sequence of preconditions, activities, and intermediate outcomes that is expected to lead to a particular longer term outcome. Developing a ToC involves critical discussion involving a range of stakeholders on the following elements:

- the project context, including the social, political and environmental conditions and other organisations able to influence change;
- the articulation of the long-term change that the project seeks to support and who should ultimately benefit from this change;
- the process or sequence of change that is anticipated in order to create the conditions for the desired long-term outcome; and
- the assumptions about how these changes happen.

The results of the discussion are generally captured in a flow chart and narrative summary.

The idea itself is reasonably simple. What makes theory of change complicated or challenging is the complexity of the social problems the project seeks to address and the environment in which the project is based. A benefit of using theory of change in evaluation is that it enables failure of theory (the expected intervention did not work out) to be differentiated from a failure of implementation (the idea was right but the intervention did not operate as planned) (Hall and Hall 2004).

As discussed in Chapter 1, the use of theory of change in youth and community work can be problematic as it involves creating 'outcome chains' that identify broad causal links between interventions and outcomes. Youth work interventions are complex, they work with individuals and groups in many different ways and no single cause can be attributed to a particular outcome. In many cases outcomes are crafted through an accumulation of different interventions. Furthermore, change is a *process* rather than an organised sequence of steps. This can make it very hard to plot a theory of change using traditional outcomes chains.

Secondly, and importantly, the process of engagement and building trust, while not an outcome in itself, is a fundamental part of the youth and community work process that needs to be captured and represented. Understanding the enabling steps that need to be taken to positively engage young people in a programme is essential in bringing about effective change. However, the 'process' aspect is neglected in many outcome chains. Arguably then, for theory of change to be beneficial in youth and community work, it needs to reflect the importance of the youth work process.

Noble and Hodgson (2014), working with the Youth Justice Board, developed an approach to address these concerns which builds the theory of change around the service-user's anticipated journey through a programme (see Figure 8.1). This model depicts an engagement or change process running through the middle with activities and outcomes on either side. This illustrates the fact that progress at each stage is influenced by both the associated activities and the process. This model better reflects the reality of change in that it shows the gradual achievement across all outcomes that happen throughout the journey, rather than one thing happening

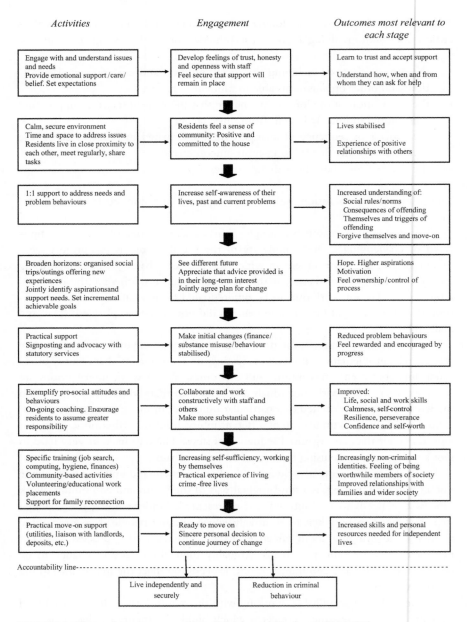

FIGURE 8.1 Illustrative outcomes chain (Noble and Hodgson 2014: 21)

and then the next. It also takes account of the fact that a young person's progress can go backwards as well as forwards.

The process of thinking about change and how it is achieved supports the development and communication of a shared understanding. This can sharpen the focus of the project's activity. Developing a shared understanding and a common language between stakeholders is essential to ensuring that the contribution that youth work makes to the improvements in outcomes for young people, is recognised and valued. A project's theory of change can help with planning how best to evaluate the effectiveness of programmes, as it provides a coherent framework for tracking whether an intervention is working as planned and how it can be improved. It can also support an organisation to be realistic about what they can reasonably offer and help them to concisely explain to funders what it is that they do.

How you approach the theory of change process and how you represent it will depend on a number of factors:

- *Purpose*
  Theory of change has a number of benefits; the importance or relevance of these will be project-specific. Developing a ToC involves identifying different views and assumptions about what the project is aiming for and how this can be achieved. This developmental process can be experienced as motivating as stakeholders will feel involved and see how their work contributes to long-term goals of the project. Developing a ToC promotes a focus on the intermediate outcomes and the articulation and assessment of these, acknowledging that change is incremental. It encourages engagement with evidence (research or practice-based) and seeks to open to scrutiny the hidden assumptions that underpin practice.
- *Size and complexity of the programme*
  Theory of change can be used at organisational, project or case level. It is easier to create a theory of change for simpler programmes and perhaps advisable to start on something small and relatively simple before moving on to the wider organisation in order to develop the necessary skills and understanding.
- *Stakeholder engagement*
  Developing a theory of change is not an individual pursuit; it must involve a range of stakeholders in a collaborative process. Who is involved and how many, again, will be project-specific. It does not need to involve everyone but should include the programme managers, staff and beneficiaries. It may also include others such as partner organisations, funders, or wider community representation. The nature of engagement can vary. It may be that the whole group is involved in workshop activity or it may be that smaller group discussions are held and work is completed outside of this to develop the flowchart and narrative for further review. Whichever process is followed it is vital that it is appropriate to the level of understanding and is inclusive.

Finally it is important to note that a theory of change will never be perfect, it should be seen as a working document that is likely to be further developed as a result of reflection and changing situations. The main aim is to produce something that everyone broadly agrees with and is useful.

Considering ethics

Ethics are the moral principles and values that guide our behaviour and decisions. It is imperative that ethical issues are considered during the formulation of the evaluation plan. In most countries, youth and community work is informed by a set of ethical principles (see Introduction). In England these are as follows:

1. Treat young people with respect, valuing each individual and avoiding negative discrimination.
2. Respect and promote young people's rights to make their own decisions and choices, unless the welfare or legitimate interests of themselves or others are seriously threatened.
3. Promote and ensure the welfare and safety of young people, while permitting them to learn through undertaking challenging educational activities.
4. Contribute towards the promotion of social justice for young people and in society generally, through encouraging respect for difference and diversity and challenging discrimination. (NYA 2000)

There are clear parallels between youth and community work practice and participatory evaluation. Batsleer (2010) identifies a number of these, including the use of groupwork, the voluntary relationship, the need for trustworthiness, the importance of sensitivity and the commitment to empowerment. As such, the ethical guidelines governing youth and community workers' everyday practice will also guide their evaluation work.

Evaluation, as a distinct discipline is also guided by ethical principles. Country-based and regional-based associations have produced guidelines for evaluators, for example, the American Evaluation Association, the Australasian Evaluation Society and the United Kingdom Evaluation Society. These are in the form of good practice guidelines, offering a set of principles that have been developed collaboratively over time. They are not seen as definitive but rather as working documents that will continue to evolve.

Ethics highlight issues of:

- benefits and risks;
- informed consent;
- anonymity and confidentiality; and
- responsibilities of evaluators to act with integrity.

Benefits and risks

This involves a consideration of any prospective benefits and reasonably foreseeable risks to participants in the evaluation; this includes all stakeholders. To begin with, this requires the purpose of the evaluation to be clearly articulated and a consideration of who will benefit from participating in the evaluation and how. The risk factors include any potential adverse effects that might arise from participating in the evaluation; these must be made explicit as they may influence willingness to participate. Adverse effects can be both physical and/or psychological, for example, stress, anxiety, diminishing self-esteem or an invasion of privacy. The aim is to ensure that the evaluation process does not harm participants in any way. However, in recognition that this can never be guaranteed, participants should be given information about additional support available in the event that they experience distress in any way during their participation.

Informed consent

Informed consent means that the person participating in the evaluation is fully informed about the evaluation being conducted. They need to be made aware of the purpose of the evaluation, informed about any potential adverse impacts of their participation, and how the evaluation findings will be used. The main purpose is that each participant is able to make an informed decision as to whether they will participate in the evaluation or not. This raises questions about whether young people themselves can give consent, and there is no universal agreement on this matter. In England, the question of whether a young person is able to give consent relates to whether they are considered mature enough to make decisions. The Fraser guidelines are used to balance their rights and wishes with the responsibility to keep them safe from harm. The Fraser guidelines originate from a legal case which looked specifically at whether doctors should be able to give contraceptive advice or treatment to under 16-year-olds without parental consent. Since then, they have been more widely used to help assess whether a young person has the maturity to make their own decisions and to understand the implications of those decisions. In contexts where young people are not legally able to give consent to participate, a parent or legal guardian must sign a consent form on their behalf. In this case it is still necessary to obtain the young person's assent to ensure their voluntary participation.

It is vitally important that gaining informed consent is not just seen as having a signed consent form. There needs to be a commitment to ensure that participants understand the nature and purpose of the evaluation as well as any potential risks and benefits for them. The consent process does not end once a form is signed but continues throughout the evaluation. Consent can be withdrawn at any time and participants must be made aware that they are free to withdraw their participation without this negatively impacting on any future involvement with the project or their relationships with the youth workers. This supports the voluntary nature of their participation in the evaluation and reduces the risk of coercion.

Anonymity and confidentiality

Participants should be assured of their anonymity and confidentiality; this often involves ensuring that their names and any information they provide that could identify them, is not disclosed in the process or the dissemination of the findings. Anonymity and confidentiality should be discussed with participants during the informed consent process, and this will involve being clear about the parameters of both. Maintaining anonymity in a participatory evaluation process can be very challenging because of its nature. Often the evaluations will be in community-based settings where participants may be well-known to each other and anonymising data may not, in itself, guarantee anonymity. This requires consideration during the planning stage and open discussion among stakeholders about their role and responsibilities in this regard. Confidentiality can also be problematic when working with young people, absolute confidentially cannot be assured. The limitations of confidentiality and when confidentiality would need to be broken, for example, for the purpose of safeguarding, must be made explicit to the participants from the outset.

Participatory evaluations often involve relatively small numbers in peer-based programmes. It is important, therefore, to consider how reports are worded to ensure there is no opportunity for people to be identified even though names are not used. What is less problematic (in terms of protecting anonymity and confidentiality) is the commitment to having a protocol in place regarding who will have access to evaluation data, while planning appropriate methods of data storage, analysis and dissemination.

Evaluator integrity

Evaluators' work should reflect four standards; utility, feasibility, propriety and accuracy. In terms of utility, the evaluator needs to ensure the evaluation addresses important questions, provides clear and understandable results and includes meaningful recommendations. Evaluations should be realistic and practical, completed in a timely and cost-efficient manner and conform to conventionally accepted standards of behaviour and ethics. Data should be collected, analysed, interpreted and reported accurately and fairly.

The 'problem' of ethics in participatory evaluation

It can be argued that participatory evaluation approaches are more ethically-aware because they take greater account of issues of power, rights and responsibilities and the role of stakeholders. They are, in essence, more egalitarian and democratic. As a consequence of this, however, they do raise some distinct ethical challenges, for example, decisions about who 'represents' the stakeholder groups, issues of power in and between stakeholders and between stakeholders and evaluators. The blurred boundaries between the evaluator and the evaluated can create difficulties in maintaining anonymity and confidentiality.

A study conducted in 2011 by the Durham Community Research Team (DCRT), led by Professor Sarah Bank, identified a number of ethical challenges in community-based participatory research that can also be found in participatory evaluation. The study highlighted the openness, fluidity and unpredictability of the participatory process that creates these particular challenges. Arguing that most ethical codes for research are concerned with the individual rights of human subjects, the study raised the need for the adoption of specific ethical guidelines to assist community-based participatory researchers (and evaluators) in the UK.

Engaging stakeholders

A stakeholder is a person who has some interest in the evaluation because they are either directly or indirectly affected by the result. Stakeholders in participatory evaluations are likely to include some (or all) of the following:

- policy-maker, such as a member of the governing board;
- project manager;
- practitioners;
- primary users (those who directly benefit from the project's service, for example, young people); and
- secondary users (those who are affected by what happens to the primary user, for example parents, community members).

Gujit (2014: 3) proposes that three questions should be asked when seeking to engage stakeholders in evaluation:

1. What purpose will stakeholder participation serve in this evaluation?
2. Whose participation matters, when and why?
3. When is participation feasible?

Involving stakeholders requires a considerable time commitment and places additional demands on the evaluator. Therefore, it is essential that the ways in which stakeholders are recruited and supported are given careful consideration during the planning phase.

While it is not necessary to include all stakeholder groups, it is necessary to be able to justify who has been included and who has not. This action can help to both identify and consider the basis of any reasoning, and make transparent the balancing of essential and desirable aspects of the evaluation. For example, it may be desirable to engage 'hard to reach' stakeholders on the grounds that they are the best people to inform us about how the project can become more accessible. However, in practice, engaging these stakeholders potentially increases risk in terms of maintaining their motivation and reliability of engagement. Stakeholder diversity presents the greatest potential for learning, and for change, and yet with diversity comes differing values orientation and an increased potential for conflict. Dilemmas, such as these, need to be explored during the process of identifying stakeholders.

Prior to any recruitment activity, the degree of engagement of each stakeholder group needs to be ascertained as this will inform the respective roles and responsibilities. Engagement can occur at any stage of the evaluation process, from the evaluation design to the data collection and analysis and the reporting of the study. The type and level of stakeholder involvement will necessarily vary depending on the focus of the evaluation, for example, between a local level impact evaluation and an evaluation of policy changes (Gujit 2014). It is not necessary for each group of stakeholders to be involved in every stage of the evaluation. However, it is essential that everyone involved understands their role and the role of others as this is fundamental to creating meaningful relationships. Approaches to recruitment may vary across the different stakeholder groups; they can include open meetings, individually targeted approaches, or specific group-targeted approaches. Whatever the approach, the aim is to clarify expectations and encourage engagement. The following areas should be included in any stakeholder recruitment activity:

- purpose and scope of evaluation;
- timescale;
- the nature of the participatory approach, including the benefits of engagement;
- stakeholders' roles and responsibilities; and
- training and support.

Equally important during any initial meetings is taking time to encourage stakeholders to raise questions, voice concerns and share ideas. Participatory evaluation is an evolving and flexible process; establishing a sense of 'working together' from the outset will significantly influence what follows. Managing stakeholder groups requires skilful facilitation, particularly in relation to developing inclusive group processes. At the beginning of any new group, members are seeking to identify whether they 'belong', what 'belonging' entails for them, and how they will be perceived by others in the group. The facilitator needs to avoid presenting themselves as being 'in control' or as being seen as the person with all the answers. Instead, they need to establish a collaborative learning stance while simultaneously demonstrating a commitment to managing the group process in relation to the interpersonal aspects of group life.

In almost every case of participatory evaluation there will be a need for training. This should be group-appropriate and designed and delivered in ways that enable and support stakeholders to meaningfully engage and fulfil their role and responsibilities. Again in line with participatory approaches, training should be strengths-based, acknowledging and building on the lived experience of the participants. An awareness of the stakeholders' knowledge and understanding of evaluation and of the project being evaluated should be used to inform any training materials. Taking account of learning styles will also help to maximise the stakeholders' engagement. Reflection is an essential aspect of evaluative skills. As such, it will be important to create opportunities to enhance reflective processes both during the training and as a part of the on-going support for stakeholders. Initially this may require more structured activity to establish a 'reflective' culture and develop skill.

Resources

It is not easy to estimate the cost of participatory evaluation. As far as possible, all the resources needed to undertake the evaluation should be identified and estimated at the outset. This should include resources that will be internally sourced as well as those that are to come from outside funding (Brophy, Snooks and Griffiths 2008). Multiple resources may be needed to support stakeholder engagement, for example, different venues, or the use of interpreters or signers. The number and type of engagement events will need to be factored in, as will any costs associated with transport, childcare and publicity materials. Additionally, participatory evaluation requires time and commitment from stakeholders and this needs to be made explicit. It is important to consider and allocate funds and resources realistically; this includes budgeting for adequate staff and stakeholder training.

In an ideal world, project evaluation will have been costed and included as part of the project implementation budget. While this is not always the case, it is now common for any grant application to require consideration and inclusion of evaluation costs. One of the criticisms of participatory evaluation is that it is costly, particularly in regards of time and, thus, at the planning stage it is necessary to clarify the requirement in terms of time, finances and other resources. The decision to use a participatory approach needs to be accompanied by an organisational commitment to appropriate resourcing. Participatory evaluation is, however, a fluid and dynamic process; it is, therefore, perhaps unrealistic to suggest that the resources required can be fully anticipated from the outset. The amount of time required in relation to supporting and mentoring a variety of stakeholders will vary, and collaborative decision-making may mean that some decisions take longer to reach agreement on than assumed.

In summary, there is much to be done prior to commencing a participatory evaluation and it is essential that sufficient time and thought is applied to the planning and preparation stage. There is a growing amount of literature available to support first-timers in their endeavours; equally, however, it must be accepted that even the best planned evaluation will likely encounter unanticipated situations, challenges and conflicts. This is not unlike the everyday practice of youth and community work and, as such, practitioners are generally well prepared to work with the dynamic nature of participatory evaluation. Gaining an organisational commitment to accept these consequences and a stakeholder commitment to strive to work to planned timescales and within existing resources can establish a shared sense of ownership and accountability.

References

Batsleer, J. (2010) 'Youth Workers as Researchers: Ethical Issues in Practitioner and Participatory Research', in S. Banks (ed.), *Ethical Issues in Youth Work* (2nd ed.), Abingdon: Routledge, pp. 178–191

Brophy, S., Snooks, H. and Griffiths, L. (2008) *Small-scale Evaluation in Health: A Practical Guide*, London, Sage Publications

Crishna, B. (2006) 'Participatory Evaluation (I) – Sharing Lessons from Fieldwork in Asia', *Child: Care, Health and Development*, Vol. 33(3), pp. 217–223

Durham Community Research Team (2011) Community-based Participatory Research: Ethical Challenges, Durham University: Centre for Social Justice and Community Action, accessed at www.ahrc.ac.uk/documents/project-reports-and-reviews/connected-communities/community-based-participatory-research-ethical-challenges/ (02.02.17)

Guijt, I. (2014) Participatory Approaches, *Methodological Briefs: Impact Evaluation 5*, UNICEF Office of Research, Florence, accessed at http://devinfolive.info/impact_evaluation/img/downloads/Participatory_Approaches_ENG.pdf (02.02.17)

Hall, I. and Hall, D. (2004) *Evaluation and Social Research*, Basingstoke: Palgrave Macmillan

Noble, J. and Hodgson, L. (2014) Theory of Change Guidance, NPC/Youth Justice Board, accessed at www.thinknpc.org/clients-and-partners/youth-justice-board/ (01.01.17)

NYA (2000) Ethical Conduct in Youth Work, Leicester: National Youth Agency, accessed at www.nya.org.uk/wp-content/uploads/2014/06/Ethical_conduct_in_Youth-Work.pdf (04.04.17)

9

DATA IN PARTICIPATORY EVALUATION

Introduction

Data refers to the information we need to address the questions we ask. Information is gathered together, usually from a variety of sources, and is analysed to produce findings that serve as the basis for the conclusions and recommendations of an evaluation. It follows then, that before any consideration of what data are needed, it is necessary to have clearly articulated the evaluation questions.

This chapter begins with a discussion about who is involved in data generation in participatory evaluation. It then moves on to examine the process of setting evaluation questions and identifying what data is needed. Two forms of data, quantitative and qualitative, are considered and the associated benefits and disadvantages of these in relation to addressing the evaluation questions are explored. This is followed by an examination of the criteria associated with the notion of trustworthiness, as applied to data generation. The chapter concludes with a summary discussion of the factors that may influence the choice of method(s) used to generate data that is both useful and appropriate in participatory evaluation.

Who 'generates' data?

A defining feature of participatory evaluation is the positioning of stakeholders as more than 'providers' of information. In the context of youth and community work, ideally these stakeholders should include young people, youth and community workers, organisational managers and representatives from the wider community in which these services are delivered. While the degree of involvement will depend on situation and context (as discussed in the previous chapter), the involvement of a range of stakeholders in decisions about what data to generate and in the generation of data is paramount.

However, the task of engaging a diverse range of stakeholders in data generation is not an easy one; any process used needs to be carefully considered in relation to accessibility and its value in supporting meaningful participation for all involved. As discussed in Chapter 4, participatory evaluation is not just about using participatory methods to generate data, but involves a rethinking about who initiates and undertakes evaluation and who benefits from it. Identifying the questions to ask about the project and the best ways to ask them, is the first step. This can be supported by taking a participatory approach to the development of the project's theory of change as discussed in the previous chapter. The process of negotiating meanings, perspectives, roles and responsibilities is time-consuming, but the benefits in terms of fostering dialogue and deliberation that contribute to a sense of shared ownership mean that this is time well spent.

What data are needed?

The response to this question will be informed by a number of factors, for example, the philosophical understanding informing the evaluation, the evaluation questions and ultimately the available resources. In participatory evaluations, forming evaluation questions is a shared process, carried out by key stakeholder groups during the planning and preparation stage. Determining what questions need to be answered is not an easy task, but it is an essential one. The general advice is to only generate data you are going to use – and use all the data you generate. However this stance is based on an assumption that we know in advance what information will be needed and useful.

Evaluation is often perceived as a logical collection of data that provides objective evidence of what works, however, it is rarely this straightforward or rational. Evaluation involves contestation and negotiation about what is valued and how. Its political nature shapes what is considered to be of value and the data used to assess this value (see Chapter 2).

Greene (1994: 534) states 'social programs ... should be evaluated according to the merit and worth of their actual effects, independent of their intended effects'. This is essential for those seeking to evaluate youth and community work. If evaluations are to capture the indirect and unintended consequences of a project's activities, then pre-defined outcomes and unanticipated outcomes need to be given equal value and attention. It will be necessary to identify data to evidence these two types of outcomes. Importantly, participatory evaluation promotes the inclusion of stakeholders in discussions about data as they are ideally placed to identify the actual benefits (both predefined and unanticipated) of the project.

Before embarking on the process of generating data it is beneficial to engage stakeholders in discussion about what 'evidence' will be accepted in answering the evaluation questions. This will necessitate establishing a shared philosophical understanding of what constitutes knowledge. Participatory evaluation is underpinned by the interpretivist paradigm in which knowledge is seen as multifaceted; as being created from 'multiple constructed realities' (see Chapter 1). Knowledge is not a 'concrete' thing that is already formed and waiting to be discovered, it is constructed through interaction. Establishing a shared understanding of what constitutes credible evidence in participatory evaluation from the outset will support the overall credibility of the evaluation findings. Policy-makers, funders and other stakeholders may doubt the credibility of evaluations that are based on alternative paradigms, given the dominance of the quasi-experimental paradigm. It is necessary and important, therefore, to educate stakeholders about the credibility of a participatory evaluation design. What 'counts' as evidence is discussed in Chapter 2 and the Bond Principles (see Table 9.1), were proposed as a useful and appropriate guide when thinking about how evidence will be generated using participatory evaluation in the context of youth and community work.

Quantitative and qualitative data

Quantitative data relate to things that can be counted and measured; they provide a numerical description. For example, the evaluation may count the number of people involved in a project activity, the number of workshops provided, or the percentage of young people involved in anti-social behaviour. Quantitative data tells us about the 'what' of the programme and tend to be collected using a systematic standardised approach and methods such as structured questionnaires or surveys. The advantages of quantitative approaches include the fact that they are often more time- and resource-efficient, they are standardised so comparisons can be easily made and the size of the effect can usually be measured. However, quantitative data is limited in their capacity to explain similarities and unexpected differences and in their ability to take account of complex environments.

Qualitative data generally take the form of words or narratives. They describe, in detail, the experience of stakeholders. For example, qualitative data can relate a service-user's experience of receiving a particular intervention, describe how a particular change came about, or what it may mean to the people involved. Qualitative data tell us about the 'how' and 'why' of a programme and tend to

TABLE 9.1 The Bond Principles

Voice and inclusion	The perspective of service-users are included in the evidence and a clear picture of who is affected and how is provided.
Appropriateness	The evidence is generated using methods that are justifiable given the nature and purpose of the evaluation.
Triangulation	The evidence has been generated using a mix of methods, data sources and perspectives.
Contribution	The evidence explores how change happens and the contribution of the intervention and factors outside of the intervention in explaining change.
Transparency	The evidence discloses the details of the data sources and methods used, the results achieved and any limitations in the data or conclusions.

be generated using less structured approaches and methods such as focus groups, group discussions and interviews. Qualitative approaches can be very effective at getting 'inside' the programme to really understand how and why it works. They are particularly useful for exploring the effects and unintended consequences of a programme and for taking account of context; however, they can be expensive and time consuming to implement. Additionally, the findings cannot be generalised to participants outside of the programme, they are context-specific and only relate to the group involved.

Chambers (2007) notes that the value of 'precision in meaning' gained through qualitative data is often contrasted with the value of 'accuracy in measurement' gained through quantitative data. This can be seen as a trade-off between breadth and depth, and between generalisability and targeting to specific, and often very small populations. For example, a sample survey of young people who participated in an alcohol awareness programme can provide representative and broadly gener-alisable information about the proportion of participants who subsequently reduced their alcohol consumption. It can tell us how this proportion differs by gender or age. However, it can only provide limited reasons for this difference. On the other hand, conducting focus groups with small groups of male and female young people will provide much richer information about differences in relation to gender or age, and the ways in which the programme changed attitudes. However, the extent to which these findings can be applied beyond the specific individuals included in the groups is limited.

There is a growing consensus that evaluation designs should incorporate both qualitative and quantitative data whenever possible, for example, the WKKF Evaluation Handbook (2004: 70) argues that 'Just as no single treatment/program design can solve complex social problems, no single evaluation method can docu-ment and explain the complexity and richness of a project.' The NSF Handbook (Frechtling 2002: 48) states 'The evaluator should attempt to obtain the most useful information to answer the critical questions about the project and, in so doing, rely on a mixed-methods approach whenever possible'. Some will remain sceptical about 'counting the uncountable' and about the appropriateness of numerical description in participatory evaluation; however, as Chambers (2009) points out, participatory methods can be used to generate numbers which can be commensurable with other non-participatory methods. He argues that 'through judgement, estimation, and expressing values, people quantify the qualitative' (Chambers 2009: 245).

Issues of trustworthiness in participatory evaluation

The trustworthiness of all forms of evaluation is important. Experimental evalu-ations are generally judged in relation to validity, generalisability, reliability and objectivity. The trustworthiness of participatory evaluation is often questioned on the grounds that it does not stand up to scrutiny against these judgement criteria. However, the argument is that these criteria are inappropriate for participatory

TABLE 9.2 Trustworthiness criteria for participatory evaluation

Positivist criteria	Interpretivist criteria
Internal validity	Credibility
External validity/generalisability	Transferability
Reliability	Dependability
Objectivity	Confirmability

evaluation as it is underpinned by an interpretivist paradigm. Instead, the trustworthiness of participatory evaluation should be judged against a different set of criteria, namely credibility, transferability, dependability and confirmability (see Table 9.2).

Internal validity is concerned with the extent to which the data measure what they purport to measure and the degree to which they provide sufficient evidence for the conclusions made by an evaluation. It raises questions about the degree to which the chosen method of data collection measures what it claims to measure. Credibility, on the other hand, involves ensuring that the methods of data generation are the most credible for the evaluation purpose. Credibility can be increased by using more than one method, as the findings can then be compared and confirmed. A number of techniques can be employed to gauge the accuracy of the findings, for example, data triangulation, triangulation through multiple analysts and 'member checks'. This sits well with participatory evaluation as a range of stakeholders are involved, to varying degrees, in the design, data generation and data analysis processes. Arguably it is the participants and the audience who can reasonably judge the credibility of the evaluation results.

External validity is concerned with the extent to which the findings of one evaluation can be applied to other situations. However, participatory evaluations are generally small-scale and programme-specific and as such it is impossible to demonstrate that the findings and conclusions are applicable to other situations and populations. The concept of transferability is used instead. The premise is that if practitioners believe their situations to be similar to that described in the evaluation, they may be able to relate the findings to their own positions (Bassey 1985). An evaluation report must be sufficiently detailed to allow readers to gain as full an understanding of the project and findings as possible. This will enable them to determine how confident they can be in transferring the findings presented in the report to their own situations.

Reliability deals with consistency and asks whether the data collection tool will provide the same information if it is administered at different times or in different places. This is problematic in participatory evaluation because the idea that people's lived experience will actually be the same, or will be reported in the same way, is nonsensical. The concept of dependability is more appropriate. This rests on the premise that the processes within the evaluation should be reported in sufficient detail to enable a future evaluator to repeat the work, not necessarily to gain the same results. Credibility and dependability are closely aligned. In practice, a demonstration of the former goes some way to ensuring the latter. This can be achieved through the use of 'overlapping methods', such as the focus group and individual interview (Lincoln and Guba 1985).

Objectivity within a positive paradigm is sought through the use of instruments that are not dependent on human skill and perception. While this is appropriate within experimental evaluation, participatory evaluation seeks to involve a range of different stakeholders, often in data generation and analysis and thus this conceptualisation of objectivity is not appropriate. The concept of confirmability is arguably better suited as it informs the steps to be taken to help ensure, as far as possible, that the evaluation findings are the result of the experiences and ideas of the participants, rather than the characteristics and preferences of the evaluator. According to Miles and Huberman (1994), a key criterion for confirmability is the extent to which the evaluator admits his or her own predispositions. Critics of participatory evaluation methods argue that it is too subjective and that evaluators lose their objectivity due to their closeness to a project and the participants. The centrality of individual and collective reflection (and reflexivity) in participatory evaluation supports confirmability. It is through reflection and reflexivity that evaluators and participants reflect on their values and biases. An ongoing analysis of the impact of these values and biases on decisions made, for example, on what information is or is not collected and who is or is not heard, address concerns about bias.

Factors influencing decisions about data generation methods

There are many ways in which data can be generated. The choice of method will generally be influenced by a range of factors, for example, the resources available, issues of credibility and appropriateness and the capabilities of those involved. Resources include financial, staffing and time. There may be a range of methods that can be used to address the same questions, however, the implementation costs of these may differ. It is important to consider costs in relation to the data needed. For example, while a large survey may be quite expensive, a small survey consisting of a few straightforward questions will be less expensive but would clearly provide less data. Time constraints must also be considered; creating and piloting survey questions can take a considerable amount of time, as can activities aimed at obtaining high response rates. Qualitative methods may be even more time consuming as data generation and data analysis merge, and the emergent nature of the process often brings forth new questions as the evaluation proceeds. Using focus groups may be more or less expensive depending on numbers of participants and while this method might provide more insightful data, this will be group-specific. Using a good mix of methods can sometimes help stretch limited funds.

Different data generation methods require different skills. Some qualitative methods, (for example in-depth interviewing, observations and focus groups), require considerable skills and supervision to generate trustworthy data. Simple quantitative methods (for example small-scale, self-administered questionnaires based on yes/no or basic scale questions) require less expertise, although they may still need to be preceded by training. Large-scale complex surveys will require more skill in terms of design and data management.

In summary, the notion of data needs to be explored from the outset, and questions such as what data are needed and how these will be generated is a topic for collective discussion amongst stakeholders. This is a complex and challenging area, and will need to be facilitated in order to enable meaningful participation. Time spent on this is time well spent, as it promotes a culture of collaboration and shared learning.

There is no ideal method for generating data. Identifying the 'best' way will inevitably involve some compromise. The involvement of a range of stakeholders in the process of data generation adds further complexity. As much time and thought will need to be given to managing the collaborative processes as to the decisions about which data generation method or methods to use. Again, this effort can produce dividends in relation to developing learning for all involved.

Engaging stakeholders in discussions about data and data needs helps to create a sense of shared ownership of a project and its mission. Importantly this engagement can bring forth new ideas and understandings about how to evidence the difference youth and community work can make to the lives of young people and the communities in which they live.

References

Bassey, M. (1985) 'Pedagogic Research: On the Relative Merits of Search for Generalisation and Study of Single Events', *Oxford Review of Education*, Vol. 7(1), pp. 73–93

Chambers, R. (2009) 'So that the Poor Count More: Using Participatory Methods for Impact Evaluation', *Journal of Development Effectiveness*, Vol. 1(3), pp. 245–246

Chambers, R. (2007) *Who Counts? The Quiet Revolution of Participation and Numbers,* Working Paper 296, Brighton: The Institute of Development Studies, accessed at www.ids.ac.uk/files/Wp296.pdf (10.03.16)

Frechtling, J. (2002) The 2002 User-Friendly Handbook for Project Evaluation, The National Science Foundation, accessed at www.nsf.gov/pubs/2002/nsf02057/nsf02057.pdf (04.04.17)

Greene, J. (1994) 'Qualitative Program Evaluation: Practice and Promise', in N. Denzin and Y. Lincoln (eds), *Handbook of Qualitative Research*, London: Sage Publications, pp. 530–544

Lincoln, Y. and Guba, E. (1985) *Naturalistic Inquiry*, London: Sage Publications

Miles, M. and Huberman, A. (1994) *Qualitative Data Analysis: An Expanded Sourcebook*, (2nd ed.), London: Sage Publications

W.K. Kellogg Foundation (2004) Evaluation Handbook, accessed at www.wkkf.org (04.04.17)

10

METHODS FOR GENERATING DATA

Introduction

In this chapter a range of methods most usually associated with participatory evaluation are explored. These include questionnaires, interviews, observation and story-telling. Each method is examined in terms of its process, the type of data it generates and the advantages and disadvantages associated with its use. A consideration of a number of factors will inform decisions about which method to use. These include the purpose of the evaluation, the participants with whom the data are generated, the resources available and the degree to which the method will intrude in or detract from the project's activities.

In deciding which method is most appropriate in any given evaluation it may be useful to explore the following questions:

- Is this method the most appropriate for the evaluation purpose?
- Will it generate usable data?
- Is this method suitable for the participants and the programme being evaluated?
- Can this method detect salient issues, meaningful changes and the various outcomes of the project?
- Is there sufficient expertise to implement this method (either available from project staff, stakeholders or an external evaluator)?

Essentially, the methods for data generation need to be the most credible for the evaluation purpose within the resources available. There is a wide array of data generation methods and tools available, some of which have been specifically designed for young people. All methods and tools have associated advantages and disadvantages. Rather than trying to provide comprehensive coverage of all possible methods, this chapter focuses on data generation methods more commonly used in participatory evaluation.

Questionnaires

Questionnaires can be used to generate both quantitative and qualitative data depending on the question type. There are two types of questions: closed questions and open questions. Closed questions generate quantitative data and generally use one of four scales; nominal, ordinal, interval and ratio. Nominal scales involve categories that have no numerical values, they are a two-point dichotomous scale that present options that are opposite each other, for example, yes/no, fair/unfair, male/female.

Both ordinal and interval scales are used to measure attitudes and behaviours rather than seeking simple yes/no responses. Ordinal scales ask the respondent to rate something, generally using a 1–5 scale. For example, an ordinal scale question asks the respondent to rank the importance of a list of qualities or activities using numbers 1 to 5 with 1 being the most important. Interval scale questions use answer choices that range from one extreme to the other (always, very often, fairly often, sometimes, almost never, never) and allow for degrees of opinion to be ascertained. In some cases, imagery is used, such as expressive faces (overjoyed, smiley, neutral, disappointed, depressed). The Likert Scale is a well-known example of an interval scale. Finally, ratio scales ask respondents for a number in response to a question, for example, how old they are, how many hours a day do they spend on social media or the number of times they visited the project in the last month.

Open questions seek to generate more insight into how the respondent feels and provide space for the respondent to express a view or opinion in their own words. This type of question generates qualitative data that tell us something about people's understandings, experiences and sense-making activities. In most cases, questionnaires will include a combination of closed and open questions.

Designing a questionnaire can be challenging; this is particularly so when it is aimed at generating data with young people. The format and the language used needs to be appropriate and unambiguous, particularly if the questionnaire is to be self-administered (young people complete the questionnaire alone). Alternatively, questionnaires can be interview-based; in these cases the evaluator is on hand to guide the young person through the questionnaire, and assistance may include reading out the questions (Heath, Brooks, Cleaver and Ireland 2009). In participatory evaluation, stakeholders can be involved in the questionnaire design, and although this may be time-consuming, it can be very useful in terms of ensuring the questionnaire is culturally relevant. It is also beneficial to pilot a questionnaire as this process generally provides invaluable feedback about the clarity and appropriateness of the questions and whether the questionnaire is user-friendly.

The advantages associated with the use of questionnaires include the ability to generate data from a large population. They can be less costly in relation to other methods and can provide anonymity for respondents. When questionnaires are self-administered, they allow respondents to take time to consider their responses and this potentially leads to better quality data. The most common disadvantage associated with questionnaires is the poor response rate. Simple and quick questionnaires may have a higher response rate. However, over-simplifying and standardising questionnaires reduces opportunities to 'dig deeper' and this can limit the data quality in comparison to some other forms of data generation. Another disadvantage arises from differences in interpretations; in other words, people may interpret each question differently. Responses are based on the reader's own interpretation of the question and this level of subjectivity is often overlooked. Further, it is not possible to judge how truthful a respondent is being, nor how seriously they have considered the questions. Finally, there is a level of 'evaluator imposition', in other words, in the development of the questionnaire the evaluator's decisions and assumptions as to what is and is not important are imposed. In participatory evaluations, this is reduced by the inclusion of other stakeholders in the focus and design of the questions, although it can never be completely eliminated.

Interviews

Interviews are a popular form of data generation in participatory evaluation as they enable the exploration of complex social and political processes, such as why and how change has occurred. They can generate rich qualitative data. There are essentially three types of interviews (structured, semi-structured and unstructured), all of which can be conducted with individuals or with groups.

Structured interviews can be understood as 'verbally administered questionnaires', the questioning is standardised in that the ordering and phrasing of the questions is consistent from interview to interview. This structuring aims to generate data that is comparable across participants; however, it does assume that a fixed sequence of questions is suitable or appropriate to all. Pre-determined questions are asked, with little or no variation and with no scope for follow-up questions to responses that warrant further elaboration. This type of interview can be seen as being informed by a traditional perception of interviews as an objective and neutral process, and while it may have a place, it is not the type generally used in participatory evaluation.

This traditional view of interviewing has been challenged; Fontana and Frey (2005) assert that interviewing is not merely the neutral asking and answering of questions but rather a process between two people whose exchanges lead to a collaborative outcome. Kvale and Brinkmann (2009) use the term 'inter-view' in recognition that knowledge is constructed in the inter-action between interviewer and interviewee, and describe the research interview as a conversation with structure and purpose. Semi-structured interviews align with this thinking as both the interviewer and the interviewee are active participants. The interviewer identifies the broad areas to be covered and creates a list of open-ended questions to be used during the conversation. This 'interview guide' is followed to promote the flow of the interview but the interviewer can pick up on themes that arise in the conversation and seek elaboration as and when they feel it is appropriate. Equally, interviewees can introduce topics that are important to them (Silverman 1993). Semi-structured interviews are a valuable data generation method because they are seen to enable interviewees to use their own unique ways of defining their world. They do, however, require a greater level of skill than structured interviews.

In unstructured interviews, no guide is used and no predetermined questions are created although the interviewer will have a clear plan in mind regarding the focus and goal of the interview. Instead, the focus is on building rapport with the interviewee and providing a conversational space to address the issues that the interviewee sees as relevant (Gibson and Brown 2009). An unstructured interview will usually begin with an open question such as 'Can you tell me about your experience of coming to this project?' and progression is based, primarily, on the initial response. Any questions posed by the interviewer will be open-ended and control over the responses is minimised. Unstructured interviews are very time-consuming; they can last for several hours and be difficult to conduct as participants (and indeed interviewers) may be unsure of what to talk about because of the lack of predetermined interview questions. The lack of control over direction, and thus data generated, can also be seen as a disadvantage, and as such, unstructured interviews are rarely used in evaluations.

Individual and group interviews

The decision about whether to use individual interviews or group interviews must be informed by the context, the topic, the preference of participants and the skill level of the interviewer. Some people may be more confident and comfortable being interviewed in a group; others may feel inhibited and anxious in group settings. Often both approaches are used; for example, a group interview may be used to generate themes that are then used to guide individual interviews, and equally data generated though individual interviews can be used as a basis for group discussion. Morgan (1997: 6) describes group interviewing as 'a research technique that collects data through group interaction on a topic determined by the researcher'. Kamberelis and Dimitriadis (2005: 887) use the term 'collective conversations' and this is useful in describing how group interviews are generally seen in participatory evaluation.

As with every other method of data generation there are a number of advantages and disadvantages associated with the use of individual and groups interviews. In terms of resources, individual interviews require more interviewer-time, but can be more easily recorded whereas group interviews are more time-efficient for the interviewer but can be difficult to record. Group interviews can also be more challenging in terms of organisation and logistics, providing less time for each participant to share their views and less control for the interviewer.

Individual interviews provide opportunities for in-depth focus on the perspectives of the interviewees, however, this focus may feel uncomfortable, especially for young people. This can lead to the young person trying to provide the 'right answer' rather than expressing their opinion or relaying their experience. Alternatively, young people may prefer the privacy of the one-to-one setting and may feel able to share more sensitive information. In group interviews the role of the interviewer is decentralised and the group setting can reduce the power differential between evaluator and participants. The interaction between participants allows for clarification, challenge, conformation, extension and shared learning. However, there can be a tendency to conformity in group settings and this may mean that some participants withhold comments that they might make in private. Group interviewing also raises challenges in terms of anonymity. The interviewer's role is to create a permissive atmosphere for the expression of personal and conflicting viewpoints (Kvale and Brinkmann 2009), and hence group work skills are essential.

A key advantage to using group interviews is that they can enable a collaborative approach to data generation; this is probably one of the most important advantages in relation to participatory evaluation. The interactions in the group, in particular the way in which participants make comparison between their opinion and the opinions of others, can provide valuable insights into complex behaviours and motivations that are not possible to access through individual interviews (Morgan 1997). The group setting is more naturalistic than the individual interview, because participants are influencing and influenced by others just as they are in real life (Krueger 1994). As a result, participants may be more open and share insights that would not be gained through individual interviews. Participants react to and build on the responses of others, producing data that is 'cumulative and elaborative' (Fontana and Frey 2005). Additionally, accounts may be more accurate as participants must defend their statements to their peers (Eder and Fingerson 2003).

Observation

Observation is a widely used means of data generation, and it involves more than 'just looking' in that it entails looking and recording systematically. Observation offers an evaluator the opportunity to gather 'live' data from naturalistic situations, in other words, the evaluator can look directly at what is taking place in situ rather than relying on second-hand accounts gained through interviews. Thus, observation has the potential to yield more valid or authentic data than would otherwise be the case with mediated or inferential methods (Cohen, Manion and Morrison 2013).

Observation is a highly flexible method that can be used to generate a wide range of data, for example, about:

- people (the characteristics of groups or individuals, power relations);
- behaviours (particularly reactions that take place);
- interactions (level of participation, level of cooperation, decision-making);
- settings (resources and their organisation, pedagogic styles, curricula); and
- routines (what happens, when and how, formal and informal).

These data can provide insights into the differences, behaviours and interactions of the participants. Observation can illuminate participants' subconscious actions that are not identifiable through other methods that focus on participants' perceptions. Additionally, insights into the programme's context, environment and activities, gained through observation, can be useful for providing the contextual information needed to frame an evaluation. A further strength is that observation may enable access and potentially, learning about sensitive issues that participants may be unwilling to talk about.

There are, of course, limitations. It is argued that the very act of observing can affect what is observed, and Patton (2011: 134) suggests this is especially the case for evaluation in the current context of 'what gets measured gets done'. Explaining the purpose and nature of the observation and seeking permission from those being observed can help to reduce the impact of the observer effect. Observer bias can also be seen as a limitation in relation to decisions about what, why, when, where, and who is being observing. Cohen et al. (2013: 459) note that 'Observations are inevitably selective, and, in part, depend as much on the observer's attention and opportunity to observe as they do on the observational instruments and data collection techniques used.' A commitment to reflexivity is required for this form of data generation. A further criticism is that observation is unable to capture the thinking that underlies the observed actions. For this reason, observations are generally used alongside other methods that seek insight into this thinking. Finally, there are resource issues; observations can be time-consuming as multiple observations are usually required to gain a representative picture of a programme, and prior knowledge of the project and its culture is necessary if the observer is to make sense of the context of evaluation in a limited amount of time.

Different formats: highly-structured, semi-structured and unstructured observations

Observations can take different forms. Highly-structured observations generate quantitative data in the form of a numerical summary of the presence or frequency of a range of predetermined incidences. Generated data are used to either support or refute a preconceived theory. In other words, it can be seen as a 'looking for' process; the observer will know in advance what they are looking for and will use a checklist of observation categories designed in advance to record the observation.

An unstructured observation does not have predetermined observation criteria; the act of observing seeks to be more inclusive and the observer works in a more iterative way. The observer will observe what is taking place before deciding on its relevance for the evaluation. When conducting a semi-structured observation, the observer will have an agenda in terms of a number of aspects or issues they seek to observe but the process of data generation to illuminate these will be far less predetermined than in the highly structured format. Observing what does not happen in a given situation may be as important for the evaluation as observing what does happen.

While both the semi-structured and unstructured format allow for issues to emerge from the observation, in most cases it is likely that the semi-structured format will provide the most useful data for a participatory evaluation context. Semi-structured and unstructured observations are generally recorded as a narrative, descriptive text, usually through the use of field notes that can be either produced during or after the observation. Observations can also be videoed, as long as this is not too intrusive, as this will provide a good record of the physical environment and the activities and interactions taking place in it.

Story-telling

The growth in popularity of story-telling as a method of generating evaluation data has been driven by a desire to secure more authentic information about complex interventions. Personal stories provide glimpses into individual and group experience and story-telling offers a powerful means to obtain information on a project's outcomes from participants' viewpoints. It can highlight both the strengths and weaknesses of a project, as well as any unintended consequences. McClintock (2003) highlights the value of story-telling in evaluations that aim for transformation:

- It relies on people to make sense of their own experiences and environments, and as such supports the change process.
- Stories can focus on particular interventions and reflect on the contextual factors that influence the outcomes of interventions.
- Stories can be analysed using existing conceptual frameworks (apriori themes) or assessed for emergent themes.

While there are similarities between unstructured interviewing and story-telling, the main difference is in the way story-telling can enable learning for participants and organisations 'in the moment' (Cooper 2014b). Story-telling can be seen as a means of 'sense making' for both the story-teller and the listener. Engaging in story-telling requires participants to look back (reflect) and look forward (imagining alternatives). Personal and social learning can be achieved through this process.

McDrury and Alterio (2003) offer a five-stage story-telling process to facilitate learning through story-telling that applies well to story-telling in participatory evaluation:

1. *Story finding*: This 'tuning in' stage involves the evaluator considering which participants have a story to tell that will support the evaluation aim and then facilitating the story-teller to consider the story they want to tell.
2. *Story telling*: This is a 'describing and deconstruction' stage. The teller is encouraged to think about their feelings and to self-question as they begin to make initial sense of their experience.
3. *Story expanding*: In this 'meaning-making' stage, the teller is facilitated to reflect more deeply through critical and probing questions.

4. *Story processing*: In this stage, the teller and the listener engage in a process that involves questioning assumptions and taken-for-granted knowledge that underpin perspectives and worldviews.
5. *Story reconstructing*: This final deliberative stage focuses on imagining alternatives, and how things might be different in the future.

The use of story-telling as a means of generating data in participatory evaluation is growing.

Two examples, the Most Significant Change (MSC) technique (Davies 1996) and Transformative Evaluation (Cooper 2014b) have already been discussed (see Chapter 6). In the context of MSC, stories are the personal accounts of change told by individuals affected by programme interventions. In Transformative Evaluation, stories are co-authored accounts by young people and practitioners. A further example is the story-telling workshop, developed in the UK by the 'In Defence of Youth Work' (IDYW) campaign. As an alternative to the dominant quantitative approach to the monitoring and evaluation of youth work, IDYW set out to encourage youth work practitioners to account for youth work through the generation of 'coal-face' stories of practice. In workshops settings, small groups of workers support each other to articulate and then interrogate a piece of their practice which, for them, best answered the question 'how does youth work achieve its special impact on young people and their lives?' Anonymised stories have been published and made available online (IDYW 2012).

Different story-telling formats: verbal, text and image

Stories can be told through a variety of media. The majority of cases stories are told verbally, as in the examples above; however, other media may work equally as well or sometimes better depending on the circumstances. These include the use of journaling, photographs and video. In some cases a range of media are used. Diaries, photographs or videos can be seen as artefacts that then become the focus of facilitated reflective dialogue in order to process and make meaning from the text or images.

Verbal stories can be generated with individuals or groups, and will need to be recorded. It is important, as far as possible, for stories to be recorded using the story-teller's own language. The 'transcripts' of the stories need to be verified by the story-teller to ensure authenticity. Pseudonyms are usually used to protect the privacy of the story-teller.

Diaries can offer rich insights into participants' experience. Keeping a diary is an individual pursuit and thus, potentially, a diary offers an 'influence-free' perspective. Diaries, when used for data generation, can be either pre-structured or unstructured (Gibson and Brown 2009). In a pre-structured diary, the author is asked to write about pre-specified aspects, for example, a young person may be asked to record their experiences of, and actions related to feeling angry. Unstructured diaries, on the other hand, ask the author to record the things of interest and importance to them. There is an increased ethical risk associated with using journaling, especially with unstructured forms; diaries are often perceived as 'private' conversations with one's self and may include sensitive information. It is necessary to ensure attention is paid to reducing the risk and to ensuring consent throughout the process.

Stories can be told in images as well as words, for example, through photographs, videos, or story-boards. The use of photography is popular with young people, as providing a camera and asking them to record events or environments can produce powerful images for reflective discussion. Video can be used in similar ways, and video-capture has grown in popularity as a means of gathering views and opinions since the appearance of the diary booth on the TV show 'Big Brother'. Anonymity is difficult when using photographs and video, and their use needs to considered carefully.

Story-boarding offers an interesting combination of talk, text and imagery; it is a creative technique which asks participants to think about their lives in narrative terms and to set down their experience in the form of drawings. As with other forms of story-telling, it is deliberative in that it involves participants in a process of exploration, reflection and learning, and is action-orientated. Law (2012) developed a three-scene technique to focus on a significant episode in a person's life; he defines an episode as any remembered turning point.

The episode is then presented as three scenes: the opening scene, the big scene and the following scene. The technique takes the participant through three stages; remembering, showing and futuring:

- *Remembering* involves the participant recalling events and actions, identifying the turning point and what it was like after the turning point.
- *Showing* is about assembling the most important thoughts and feelings into a words-and-pictures account of the three scenes. The words and pictures portray significant people, locations, interactions, thoughts and feelings.
- *Futuring* is about identifying what action can now be taken to move things on.

Storytelling as a means of generating data has a number of strengths in the context of participatory evaluation. It is, by its nature, a participatory and collaborative process which has a focus on learning for all and it accommodates values and respects diverse ways of knowing and learning. Stories enable us to gain insight into the lived experience of young people, and allow us to understand the degree of their success in achieving expected outcomes as well as identifying unexpected outcomes and unintended consequences in ways that other methods may not. A further strength is that people enjoy the storytelling process (Dart and Davies 2003) and the stories themselves can enhance one's sense of self (Cooper 2014a).

Sole and Wilson (2002) identify a range of benefits that story-telling offers in relation to organisational learning. They argue that sharing experiences through story-telling enables the development of shared norms and values. Story-telling builds trust as it requires people to open up to others in relation to their values, thoughts and feelings as well as their strengths and weaknesses. Importantly, for a youth and community work context, story-telling can illuminate tacit knowledge; knowledge that is embedded and embodied and which escapes many other forms of knowledge generation. This in turn can support a process of unpacking the practices and mental frames that subconsciously shape our work. Story-telling also generates emotional connectedness in a way that other methods of data generation fail to; stories 'stick' with us long after the telling. Finally, stories speak to a broad audience and the inclusion of participants' voices and perspectives can help communicate outcomes and the importance of the work to stakeholders, funders and the wider community.

There are, of course, limitations associated with story-telling as a means of generating data. A common perception of a story is that it is fiction or fantasy and this can raise credibility issues when stories are used as data. Questions may be raised as to whether stories are accurate and credible evidence as opposed to just anecdotal. Stories are essentially individual constructions of human experience and thus subjective. It is always the case that there are different stories to be told. The decision as to which story to tell rests with the individual, although this decision is open to influences; for example, who the listener is, what motivates the teller, and what is the perceived purpose of telling. Stories are also incomplete, as Stake (2005: 456) argues, 'the whole story exceeds anyone's knowing and anyone's telling'. Rather than being representative of the whole, stories are 'snapshots' of particular moments. Stories tend to highlight positive aspects and, as such, can mask poor practice or performance. They are also dependent upon skill level in regards to 'telling', but especially in regards to active listening.

In summary, the methods used to generate data should be determined by their appropriateness in addressing the evaluation purpose. They need to be able to produce data that are both useful and usable. The question of resource availability will inform decisions about method choice, including whether there are sufficient skills, training and time available. Using mixed methods and generating both qualitative and quantitative data, is seen to enhance the robustness and credibility of the findings of an evaluation. In the context of youth and community work, using data generation methods which reflect the nature of youth and community work practice and which offer extended learning opportunities for participants is an important factor (see Chapter 7). Alignment between data generation methods and youth work methods adds value and increases the likelihood of sustained practitioner engagement. Finally, while four methods have been examined in this chapter, evaluators should continually explore the potential to create new and innovative methods of data generation.

References

Cohen, L., Manion, L. and Morrison, K. (2013) *Research Methods in Education* (7th ed.), Abingdon: Routledge

Cooper, S. (2014a) 'Putting Collective Reflective Dialogue at the Heart of the Evaluation Process', in *Reflective Practice*, Vol. 15(5), pp. 563–578

Cooper, S. (2014b) 'Transformative Evaluation: Organisational Learning through Participative Practice', *The Learning Organization*, Vol. 21(2), pp. 146–157

Dart, J. and Davies, R. (2003) 'A Dialogical, Story-based Evaluation Tool: The Most Significant Change Technique', in *American Journal of Evaluation*, Vol. 24(2), pp. 137–155

Davies, R. (1996) 'An Evolutionary Approach to Facilitating Organisational Learning: An Experiment by the Christian Commission for Development', in D. Mosse, J. Farrington and A. Rew (eds), *Development as Process: Concepts and Methods for Working with Complexity*, London and New York: Routledge/ODI

Eder, D. and Fingerson, L. (2003) 'Interviewing Children and Adolescents', in J. Holstein and J. Gubrium (eds), *Inside Interviewing: New Lenses, New Concerns*, London: Sage Publications, pp. 33–54

Fontana, A. and Frey, J. (2005) 'The Interview: From Neutral Stance to Political Involvement', in N. Denzin and Y. Lincoln (eds), *The Sage Handbook of Qualitative Research* (3rd ed.), London: Sage Publications, pp. 695–727

Gibson, W. and Brown, A. (2009) *Working with Qualitative Data*, London: Sage Publications

Heath, S., Brooks, R., Cleaver, E. and Ireland, E. (2009) *Researching Young People's Lives*, London: Sage Publications

IDYW (2012) This is Youth Work: Stories from Practice, accessed at https://indefenceofyouthwork.com/the-stories-project/ (11.10.16)

Kamberelis, G. and Dimitriadis, G. (2005) 'Focus Groups: Strategic Articulations of Pedagogy, Politics and Inquiry', in N. Denzin and Y. Lincoln (eds), *The Sage Handbook of Qualitative Research* (3rd ed.), London: Sage Publications, pp. 887–907

Krueger, R. (1994) *Focus Groups: A Practical Guide for Applied Research* (2nd ed.), London: Sage Publications

Kvale, S. and Brinkmann, S. (2009) *Interviews: Learning the Craft of Qualitative Research Interviewing* (2nd ed.), London: Sage Publications

Law, B. (2012) The Use of Narrative: Three-scene Storyboarding – Learning for Living, accessed at www.hihohiho.com/storyboarding/sbL4L.pdf (05.04.17)

Morgan, D. (1997) *Focus Groups for Qualitative Research* (2nd ed.), London: Sage Publications

McClintock, C. (2003) 'Using Narrative Methods to Link Program Evaluation and Organization Development', in *The Evaluation Exchange*, Vol. IX(4), accessed at www.hfrp.org/evaluation/the-evaluation-exchange/issue-archive/reflecting-on-the-past-and-future-of-evaluation/using-narrative-methods-to-link-program-evaluation-and-organization-development (21.07.16)

McDrury, J. and Alterio, M. (2003) *Learning Through Story-telling in Higher Education: Using Reflection and Experience to Improve Learning*, London: Kogan Page

Patton, M. (2011) *Developmental Evaluation: Applying Complexity Concepts to Enhance Innovation and Use*, London: Guilford Press

Silverman, D. (1993) *Interpreting Qualitative Data: Methods for Analysing Talk, Text and Interaction*, London: Sage Publications

Sole, D. and Wilson, D. (2002) Storytelling in Organizations: The Power and Traps of Using Stories to Share Knowledge in Organizations, LILA, Harvard, Graduate School of Education, accessed at https://pdfs.semanticscholar.org/b567/5890f706d7f8e1bf1dc-01f977a0e34afc421.pdf (05.04.17)

Stake, R. (2005) 'Qualitative Case Studies', in N. Denzin and Y. Lincoln (eds), *The Sage Handbook of Qualitative Research* (3rd ed.), London: Sage Publications, pp. 443–466

11
ANALYSING DATA

Introduction

It is often the case that while the generation of data is carefully considered, insufficient attention is given to the planning of and preparation for data analysis. Generating information requires a great deal of work and time; however, analysing it is perhaps the most important step in conducting an evaluation. It makes good sense to consider how the data are to be analysed before they are generated. This will help to ensure their appropriateness and usefulness.

Having generated data, the next step is to make sense of it. It can be helpful to think about this sense-making stage of the evaluation as four distinct processes (Patton 2008). These processes are analysis (what are the data telling us?), interpretation (what does this mean?), judgement (what is the value of this?) and recommendation (how can this knowledge lead to improvement?). While it is helpful to think of these processes as distinct, it is important to understand that they are interrelated. Analysis will inform interpretation and judgements will be based on both the analysis and interpretation. Recommendations will be shaped by the analysis, interpretation and judgement.

The focus of this chapter is on analysis. It begins with a discussion on the analysis of quantitative data and explains the basic use of statistics. Generally, more qualitative data than quantitative data is generated in participatory evaluation and, therefore, the chapter explores qualitative data analysis in more detail. The most common form of qualitative analysis, namely content analysis, is presented and explained using an example from a Transformative Evaluation of a youth work project.

The involvement of stakeholders in the analysis and interpretation of data is seen as beneficial, but there are challenges. Using a further example from Transformative Evaluation, the involvement of stakeholders is examined and the benefits highlighted. This chapter challenges the perspective that stakeholder engagement in analysis reduces the validity of evaluation findings, arguing that this depends on the way in which validity is perceived.

Approaches to data analysis

Put simply, the process of analysis involves the organising and explaining of generated data. There are many different approaches to analysis; the decision as to which approach to take will generally be informed by the types of evaluative questions we ask and the type of data generated to answer those questions. Searching for the perfect method of data analysis is arguably fruitless (Coffey and Atkinson 1996), however, it is clear that the approach used must be compatible with the evaluation paradigm. As most participatory evaluations will generate more qualitative than quantitative data, the emphasis in this chapter is on analysing qualitative data. These two different types of data require different approaches to analysis.

Analysing quantitative data

Large scale evaluations are likely to use commercial software packages to analyse data, but these are not appropriate and often not affordable for small-scale projects. Small-scale projects are more likely to use descriptive statistics (sometimes called 'measures of central tendency'), and frequency and/or percentage distributions. The first step of the analysis involves the tabulation of data using the different variables in the data set. This provides a comprehensive picture of what the data looks like and can assist the identification of patterns. It is important to include the total population number when presenting the analysis: this is denoted by 'n= the population size'.

A *descriptive* statistic is the result of a calculation that is used to 'describe' the data set. The most frequently used descriptive statistics are the mean, mode or median. The mean is calculated by adding together all the numbers in the set and dividing the result by the amount of numbers in the set, for example

$$25+28+31+24+30 = 138/5 = 27.6$$

When the numbers in the set are clustered around a central value as in the example above, the mean can be useful in indicating a typical score; it is representative. However, if the numbers in the set are very widely spread, very unevenly distributed or clustered around an extreme value, then the mean can be misleading as shown in the following example

$$12+15+31+21+29+19+40+1 = 168/8 = 21$$

The mode is the number that occurs most often in the data set; it can be used to indicate a 'normal' or 'usual' figure and is a useful descriptive statistic when the numbers in a distribution are not evenly spread around a central value. However, the mode is an unstable figure as a single number change can alter the mode significantly, for example, in a data set such as 1, 2, 2, 6, 7, 8, 10 the mode is 2, but in the data set 1, 2, 6, 7, 8, 10, 10 the mode is 10.

The median is the central point in a data set, to calculate this all the numbers are placed in order and the central number is identified. When there is no central number (that is, when there is an even amount of numbers) the median is calculated by adding the two central numbers and dividing by two. In contrast to the mode, the median remains relatively unaltered by an extreme number change and thus is a more representative figure. However, using the median of a set of numbers can be very time-consuming when the set is large, for example, when it contains a hundred numbers.

A *frequency distribution* is an organised tabulation of the number of individual scores located in a given category. It shows how many times something occurred or how many responses fit into a particular category, for example, 25 of the 60 participants were over 15 years of age, 15 of the 25 participants rated the workshop as 'very useful' in helping deal with family communication problems.

A *per cent distribution* shows the proportion of participants who are represented within each category, for example, 42 per cent of the participants (n=60) were over 15 years of age, 60 per cent of participants (n=25) rated the workshop as very useful in helping deal with family communication problems.

As Stake and Schwandt (2006: 414) state 'Measurement is easy. Interpreting measurement is difficult.' Interpretation involves a questioning of the numbers, for example, are answers as you expected? Do some responses look too high or too low? There is a need to check for patterns within the data set and it may be appropriate to identify any correlations between the data. A correlation is a measure of association, a statistical calculation that describes the nature of the relationship between two variables. It can be both a positive and a negative relationship. For example, positive correlation is when an increase in factor A can be seen as associated with an increase in factor B. Negative correlation is opposite of this, an increase in factor A is associated with a decrease of factor B. An important thing to remember when using correlations is that a correlation does not explain causation; it simply indicates a relationship or pattern that exists. It does not mean that one variable is the cause of the other.

Quantitative data will need to be presented and explained. Presentation is generally through the use of charts, tables and graphs as this enables the findings to be seen more clearly and quickly. It is important to accompany these with narrative summaries to effectively communicate the key findings to others.

Analysing qualitative data

Qualitative data, for example, interview transcripts, field notes, narratives and images, require a different approach to analysis. This involves looking at the content of the data and generally entails a process of identifying commonalities, relationships and differences within a data set (Marshall and Rossman 2006). The generation of

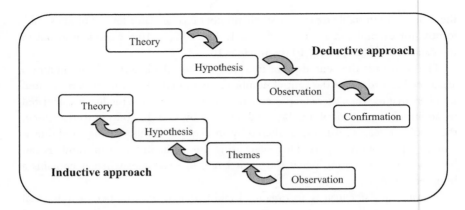

FIGURE 11.1 Deductive and inductive approaches

themes (thematic analysis) is a key aspect. Before moving on to look at content analysis in more detail, it is important to consider the two main approaches that can be taken in qualitative data analysis, namely deductive and inductive. Deductive analysis starts from the position of a preformed hypothesis and data are collected to 'test' this hypothesis. The analysis is focused by the hypothesis, and the aim is to either support or reject it. On the other hand, the inductive approach has no preformed hypothesis; the analysis involves generating theory from the data. Figure 11.1 illustrates these two approaches.

In relation to evaluation, a deductive approach can be used to test a project's 'theory of change'. This will require the theory to be broken down into more specific hypotheses that can be 'tested' with specific data and this approach can result in a 'tentative' confirmation (or not) of the project's theory of change. This approach is often aligned with outcomes evaluation. An inductive approach takes a different path, using the data to develop broader generalisations and theories. This approach is sometimes referred to as a 'bottom up' approach. The deductive approach is often aligned with process evaluation, and is regularly used in participatory evaluation.

Content analysis

Content analysis can be understood as a general term for a number of different strategies used to analyse text (Powers and Knapp 2006). Krippendorff (2013: 24) defines content analysis as 'a research technique for making replicable and valid inferences from texts (or other meaningful matter) to the contexts of their use'. He argues that it can provide new insights, increase understanding of particular phenomena and inform practice. Content analysis is often associated with quantitative analysis as a consequence of its origins where it was mainly used to analyse mass media products, for example, propaganda, newspapers or literature. This form of content analysis involved counting the frequency of predetermined categories (words or phrases).

Some researchers who favour qualitative approaches, have criticised the interpretation of content analysis as just a numerical counting exercise, arguing instead
that the focus should be on understanding the participants' categories and to see
how they are used. For Krippendorff (2013), the quantitative versus qualitative
distinction is a mistaken dichotomy; instead, he argues that both are necessary for
the analysis of text. Miles and Huberman (1994) usefully identify three concurrent
activities that take place during data analysis; these are data reduction, data display
and conclusion drawing. Qualitative approaches to enquiry can produce large data
sets, and as such there is a need to 'reduce' these to a manageable level. This is
achieved through the process of coding, based on an examination of the data for
recurrent instances of some kind. These instances are grouped together using a
coding system.

Coding data and generating themes

The first step is that of familiarisation with the data, this involves reading the data
a number of times. Through this familiarisation work, an initial understanding of
the data begins to form, and this prepares the ground for coding. Coding involves
the creation of categories that are used to describe the general features of the data.
It is through the process of coding that commonalities and differences within a data
set can be identified. Coffey and Atkinson (1996) describe coding as a conceptual
device for interrogating the data and for opening up new meaning, in other words
coding is not simply descriptive, it provides a means to relate the data to existing
understandings.

There are two types of codes; apriori and empirical. Apriori codes are defined
prior to the examination of the data and will reflect the main concerns of the evaluation. It is important to note that apriori codes will influence the data generation.
For example, they are used to shape the interview questions and inform decisions
about who is involved and the methods used. The qualitative data (for example,
interview transcripts, stories, field notes) are then examined for the presence of
these codes. The analysis may reveal that some of the apriori codes are not evident
in the transcripts to the level anticipated, and this may point to a need to revisit the
evaluation design.

The second type, empirical codes, emerge through the examination of the data.
Developing empirical codes is usually a much more time-consuming process as
code lists will need refining as more data is interrogated. However, the advantage
is that there is less risk of missing important issues and more opportunity of capturing unanticipated outcomes. Through examination and re-examination of the
data, words or phrases that are considered to be important or interesting are identified and marked, often in different colours. A descriptive name (code) is attached
to these. It is likely that too many codes will be created in the first instance, and
re-examination is required to reduce and refine the codes. The coding process leads
into the generation of themes. 'Themes' can be understood as 'super-categories'
or high-level categories that provide an overall structure to the data. They also

provide a structure for the evaluation report. As Gibson and Brown (2009: 129) state 'analysis is (...) about story-telling and as any novelist will attest, themes are a useful device for narrative construction'. Themes are generated through the process of coding, but move beyond description to interpretation. Themes 're-present' the data in terms of commonalties, differences and relationships in the context of existing understandings and, therefore, enable new conceptualisations to emerge.

Content analysis in Transformative Evaluation

Transformative Evaluation generates data in the form of a number of co-authored stories. The analysis of these stories takes place at two levels; as part of the ongoing evaluation process and, annually, as a distinct activity. The two processes are examined to provide an example of content analysis in participatory evaluation.

Transformative Evaluation is a four-stage process (see Chapter 6 for detail) and it is at stage two that the first level of analysis takes place. In this stage the youth workers bring together the stories that they generated with young people over a period of four months, usually about twenty stories. At this point, the stories are young people's narrative accounts of what they have identified as significant changes that happened for them as a result of their involvement with the youth project.

To begin the content analysis, these stories are read aloud verbatim. The youth workers then go about the task of 'grouping' the stories according to their content – in other words they identify codes to sort the twenty or so stories into four or five groups and agree through consensus how these groups should be labelled. In practice, this process is both more challenging and more time-consuming than is often expected. Identifying the most important aspect of each story is not always straightforward, nor is the identification of an appropriate label (code). It is often the case that too many codes are identified and the group need to re-visit the stories two or three times before reaching consensus.

Importantly the process of analysis supports professional learning as much as it supports the evaluation results; in fact, its value is probably more in terms of the former rather than the latter. Engaging youth workers as 'data analysts' is central to the ethos of Transformative Evaluation, and the grouping of stories and assigning of domain names leads to indepth reflection and analysis of their own practice. It generates 'collective dialogical spaces' in which workers can explore issues that they identify as important, and question some of the 'taken for granted' assumptions that exist. Being involved in the analysis enables youth workers to collectively articulate their values and beliefs and this can lead to feelings of empowerment (Cooper 2014).

The Transformative Evaluation process is usually repeated three times a year and this can generate up to seventy or eighty stories per annum. The second level of analysis involves a further content analysis of this full data set. Analysis, at this level, is likely to be facilitated by an external evaluator due to the size of the data set, but it can still be participatory if desired. Content analysis of the full data set may involve both a qualitative and quantitative approach.

Stories may be grouped using apriori codes that represent the project's planned outcomes or that reflect the project's theory of change. Each story is examined and the presence or absence of a particular code, or indeed multiple codes, is recorded. This is done by using a nominal scale (1 = presence of a code, 0 = absence of a code). Information relating to each story-teller is included, for example, their gender, age and ethnicity, as is information relating to which stage each story reached within the evaluative process (those selected by the youth workers at stage 2 and those selected by the stakeholders group at stage 3). This information is then tabulated to enable comparison and to highlight differences and relationships between variables. An extract from a code table created from a set of stories is shown in Table 11.1.

Quantitative analysis can be conducted using this code table. Descriptive statistics (mean, mode or medium) and frequency or percentage distributions can be used to provide information about the story-tellers. For example, the analysis can show the percentage of stories generated by male and female young people, and the average age of story-tellers. Cross tabulation can tell us something about what kind of stories are being selected at different stages, for example all selected stories are from young people aged twelve years and over. The data set can also be examined for correlation between codes, but again a word of warning, this does not provide causal information. Quantitative analysis, as described above, can be used to answer the 'how much' or 'how many' questions of the evaluation and may identify relationships between variables. However, it does not provide any insights in to why interventions work or do not work. In order to generate a more nuanced understanding, the stories can be subjected to further analysis using a qualitative approach to content analysis.

TABLE 11.1 An example of a code table

Story	Story-teller information			Code			
	Age	M/F	Stage	Health awareness	Employability skills	Fostering resilience	Increased confidence
1	14	F	1	1	0	1	0
2	9	M	1	0	0	0	1
3	15	M	2	0	1	0	1
4	14	M	1	1	0	1	1
5	10	M	1	0	0	1	1
6	17	M	2	1	1	0	1
7	10	M	1	1	0	1	0
8	16	F	1	0	1	0	1
9	15	F	3	1	1	1	0
10	12	F	2	1	0	0	1
11	15	F	1	0	1	1	1
12	16	F	1	1	1	0	0
13	16	M	1	0	1	0	1
14	10	F	1	1	0	1	1
15	13	M	1	1	0	0	1

A qualitative analysis involves the examination of the individual stories to indentify key characteristics (empirical codes) within them. Qualitative analysis can take longer than quantitative analysis as it will be necessary to read and re-read the data several times to identify and refine the codes. The emergent codes are then interpreted to create overarching themes. Comparisons across the stories can be made to identify differences and commonalties. This interpretive process moves away from generating information about how many young people benefitted from a project's activities towards generating new insights about what works, when and for whom. Importantly, this approach can identify unanticipated outcomes.

Involving stakeholders in data analysis

The engagement of stakeholders in the analysis and interpretation of data is an essential element of participatory evaluation. Although the level or degree may vary across evaluations, engagement in this stage is often seen as the most important in the whole evaluation process (Heath, Brooks, Cleaver and Ireland 2009). Discussions about how stakeholders can be involved needs to take place at the planning stage; however, this is sometimes overshadowed by a focus on engaging stakeholders in data generation. This is perhaps because data generation is seen as a more creative, and consequently, more engaging part of the evaluation. Analysis and interpretation has a poor image in comparison. It is often being perceived as a desk-bound activity, surrounded with piles of data and as something that can only be done by experts. These perceptions need to be challenged.

Analysis and interpretation in participatory evaluation needs to be planned and designed to fit seamlessly within the whole, not as something that happens afterwards by somebody else. The degree of stakeholder involvement will be determined by the purpose of the evaluation. For example, evaluations that have learning and improvement as central foci can prioritise participation whereas those that seek to generate 'evidence' for a policy audience will likely need to combine participatory analysis processes with externally acceptable approaches. The level of engagement can also vary. It may be appropriate for an initial analysis of data to be conducted by the evaluator, followed by early findings being presented to stakeholders, who then provide context and input on interpretation.

There are many benefits to involving stakeholders; first and foremost they can provide enormous help in analysing and interpreting data, their 'insider perspective' can bring considerable understanding and insight. They can help clarify the meaning of words or phrases and can interpret the cultural significance of particular interactions. Stakeholders' interpretations can be more context-specific and thus more meaningful (Dyson 2000). A reason often cited for not involving stakeholders, particularly young people, is that they will have no interest in this aspect of the process; this may say more about the evaluators than the stakeholders. On the contrary, engaging stakeholders enables them to see what happens with the information they provide, it can reinforce their commitment by demonstrating that their perspectives are valued and valuable. Engaging stakeholders also has the benefit of improving evaluation use, as Jackson and Kassam (1998: 1) argue:

> It is precisely by sharing the different types of knowledge they bring to the evaluation process – and the new knowledge they create together – that citizens and professionals can generate analysis that will render interventions more capable of yielding significant and lasting results.

For some, the engagement of stakeholders in analysis and interpretation is viewed as problematic based on what can be perceived as a lack of rigour. The opening up of the process to 'unskilled' participants is seen to lead to a decline in quality and credibility of the findings. Those aligned with participatory approaches strongly dispute this; Lincoln and Guba (1985: 315) argue that the process of testing data, preliminary categories and interpretations with stakeholders is 'the single most crucial technique for establishing credibility'.

The notion of objectivity has been subject to long debate:

> You cannot but help read the data through the filter of your own worldview, your own preconceptions and your own motives – and wanting to find evidence of certain events or processes in the data can be a very powerful motive. (Schreier 2012: 90)

If we accept Schreier's view it follows that analysis and interpretation of data from different perspectives can lead to more valid interpretations of the evaluation data.

In addressing the issue of skills, O'Sullivan (2004) asserts that those who believe analysis is beyond the objectivity and capacity of stakeholders should think again. As with any participatory process, the preparation and 'training' of stakeholders is essential in enabling their meaningful participation. For some, there is a tension between rigour and participation, however, this does depend on how 'rigour' is perceived. Again, this raises questions about the way in which judgements about quality are made. Participation may not support traditional measures of validity; however, if catalytic validity (the degree to which the research process has transformative or empowering outcomes) is used as the measure, then full and meaningful participation is seen as central. The engagement of stakeholders in the analysis and interpretation of data increases the likelihood that findings and recommendations will be put to practical use.

In summary, this chapter has explored approaches to data analysis, and has highlighted the benefits of engaging stakeholders in this stage of evaluation. It sets out to demystify the processes involved in order to encourage the view that, with appropriate planning and careful design, analysis and interpretation of evaluation findings can be an engaging and creative activity for all involved. It seems paradoxical that stakeholders are not more involved in the analysis of data in participatory evaluation. Why is it that they can be trusted to generate data but not perceived as capable, or as trusted to evaluate those data?

Participatory analysis is a valuable element of participatory evaluation, but it may not be appropriate in every situation. In determining the appropriateness for your evaluation, the following questions should be considered:

- In what ways might participatory analysis improve the quality of findings and recommendations?
- Will the engagement of stakeholders result in positive outcomes for stakeholders?
- Will the participatory analysis approach fit within the project timeline and available resources?

The process of analysis is bound up with issues of power and these issues need to be de-constructed to ensure that stakeholders are not excluded from this stage of evaluation. Evaluators will need to examine their own perceptions and values, and those that commission evaluations, if they claim to be working within the participatory paradigm. Attention needs to be given to developing appropriate processes which enable stakeholders to engage as fully as possible in the analysis of data.

References

Coffey, A. and Atkinson, P. (1996) *Making Sense of Qualitative Data: Complementary Research Strategies*, London: Sage Publications

Cooper, S. (2014) 'Putting Collective Reflective Dialogue at the Heart of the Evaluation Process', in *Reflective Practice: International and Multidisciplinary Perspectives*, Vol. 15(5), pp. 563–578

Dyson, S. (2000) 'Working with Sickle Cell/Thalassaemia support groups', in H. Kemshall and R. Littlechild (eds), *User Involvement and Participation in Social Care*, London: Jessica Kingsley Publishers, pp. 159–174

Gibson, W. and Brown, A. (2009) *Working with Qualitative Data*, London: Sage Publications

Heath, S., Brooks, R., Cleaver, E. and Ireland, E (2009) *Researching Young People's Lives*, London: Sage Publications

Jackson, E. and Kassam, Y. (eds) (1998) *Knowledge Shared: Participatory Evaluation in Development Cooperation*, Boulder, CO: Kumarian Press/IDRC

Krippendorff, K. (2013) *Content Analysis: An Introduction to its Methodology* (3rd ed.), London: Sage Publications

Lincoln, Y. and Guba, E. (1985) *Naturalistic Inquiry*, London: Sage Publications

Marshall, C. and Rossman, G. (2006) *Designing Qualitative Research*, London: Sage Publications

Miles, M. and Huberman, M. (1994) *Qualitative Data Analysis*, London: Sage Publications

O'Sullivan, R. (2004) *Practicing Evaluation: A Collaborative Approach*, London: Sage Publications

Patton, M. (2008) *Utilization-focused Evaluation* (4th ed.), London: Sage Publications

Powers, B. and Knapp, T. (2006) *Dictionary of Nursing Theory and Research* (3rd ed.), New York: Springer Publishing Company

Schreier, M. (2012) *Qualitative Content Analysis in Practice*, London: Sage Publications

Stake, R. and Schwandt, T. (2006) 'On Discerning Quality in Evaluation', in I. Shaw, J. Greene and M. Mark (eds), *The Sage Handbook of Evaluation*, London: Sage, pp. 404–418

12

SHARING KNOWLEDGE

Introduction

This chapter focuses on the processes used to share knowledge generated through participatory evaluation. The active, purposeful process of knowledge sharing is often overlooked and attention paid only to the production of an 'end of evaluation' report. While clearly the evaluation report is an important outcome, it is not the only means of sharing knowledge generated through evaluation. This chapter aims to encourage a wider consideration of the process of dissemination. It seeks to encourage the reader to think beyond the 'reporting back' to managers and funders in order to consider how knowledge generated through participatory evaluation can be shared with a wider audience.

Gibson and Brown (2009) assert that the presentation of evaluation findings is more than a mere representation and argue that it should be seen as an active and creative part of the evaluation process. Communicating evaluation outcomes helps to ensure that evaluation leads to an increased understanding of a project's 'theory of change' and to improvements in practice (Alkin, Christie and Rose 2006). Participatory evaluation is time-consuming and resource-heavy and as such, we should strive to maximise its value by broadening the dissemination of the knowledge it creates.

The chapter begins with a focus on voice, audience and message and raises questions as to who should be involved in communicating the evaluation findings and to whom these should be communicated. In the context of youth and community work, these are essential questions given that the practice and the value of this work is generally misunderstood and undervalued. The chapter addresses the report-writing aspect and presents some guidance in terms of report composition and format before moving to explore more participatory forms of dissemination.

The chapter concludes with an exploration of the ways in which evaluation knowledge (and skills) can be captured and shared. Participatory evaluations are shaped by those who use them and, therefore, require a commitment to interrogate the assumptions, actions and outcomes arising from them. Meta-evaluation ensures that ongoing attention is given to our evaluation practices.

Voice, audience and message

Participatory evaluation is underpinned by a commitment to democratic pluralism. It seeks to promote the inclusion of and collaboration between stakeholders and, therefore, any processes used to share knowledge generated through participatory evaluation should also be shaped by these commitments.

For those working within the participatory paradigm, it is necessary to give appropriate attention to the ways in which participants' voices are heard through the dissemination process. It simply does not make sense to involve participants in all other aspects of the evaluation and then exclude them from the knowledge-sharing process. Additionally, their involvement can help ensure maximum impact across a wider variety of audiences. While knowledge generated through evaluation is primarily used to inform decisions relating to the future direction of the project itself, it should also be used beyond this, to inform the wider development of policy and practice. As Stuart, Maynard and Rouncefield (2015: 191) state: 'Evaluators should consider not only how their evaluations support learning for young people, practitioners, projects and organisations, but also how they can promote awareness of important youth issues and inform policy change.'

Identifying your audience is of key importance and involves addressing the questions of who you are seeking to communicate with and for what purpose. It is highly likely that you will have multiple audiences and multiple purposes, for example, the funder, a range of stakeholders (internal and external), the wider communities of practice, policy-makers and academics. Alkin et al. (2006: 386) assert that 'developing as complete an understanding as possible of what audiences want to know, why they want to know it and what use they intend to make of it' supports effective communication of evaluation findings.

Communicating clearly the findings of an evaluation is not a simple task. Distilling a mass of information, deciding what is important, and presenting this in an accessible form can be challenging. It is often the case that efforts made to develop clear communication of complex issues also help to create clarity of thought. The need to communicate with a variety of audiences adds further complexity as different audiences will likely benefit from different formats and modes of communication. The following questions can be used to guide this stage of the evaluation process:

- What should be shared?
- How best can we share it?
- Are we communicating in a way that can be received and understood?
- Are we being considerate of our audience as we prepare our message?

No project is perfect; it is the responsibility of the evaluator to present as comprehensive a picture as possible. This will include the positive, unfavourable and ambiguous findings, and the particular limitations that affected these. It is important not to over-simplify or overstate evaluation findings, and care needs to be taken not to ignore the importance of context in the generation of findings. It is not uncommon for there to be some ambiguous findings, some uncertainty; this should not be hidden from view but made transparent and used positively to highlight the need for further investigation. Participatory evaluation generally generates more qualitative data than quantitative data and it can be useful to include direct quotations within the 'message'. The use of narratives and stories can provide rich description, allowing the audience to get a sense of 'what it is like to have been there' (Stake 2004: 211). This supports their ability to form judgements about the value, or shortcomings, of the project.

The most common form of communicating findings is a written report, although other forms do exist and are arguably as important for sharing knowledge generated by participatory evaluations. Patton (2008) is quite clear that an evaluation report should be considered as a means to an end in that its purpose is to promote the use of evaluation findings. The process of sharing the outcomes of the evaluation with others can lead to new insights, new questions to be asked and therefore can inform future evaluations.

Writing an evaluation report

Generally, written evaluation reports are the most common form of reporting evaluation findings. There are two forms of written evaluation reports; interim and final. Interim reports are sometimes required as part of the contractual agreement with the funder, however, even when this is not the case, they can be a useful means of sharing emerging knowledge with key stakeholders. They are often more informal than final reports in terms of format; however, this should be agreed beforehand as sometimes the expectation is that they will follow a similar format, but be briefer.

Patton (2008) argues against a standard reporting format; rather he champions a 'fit for purpose' approach to choosing a format asserting that 'the best format is the one that fulfils the purpose of the evaluation and meets the needs of specific intended users in a specific situation' (ibid.: 509). He developed a set of principles to support evaluators to create useful reports:

1. Be intentional about reporting, that is, know the purpose of the report and stay true to that purpose.
2. Stay user-focused: Focus the report on the priorities of the primary intended users.
3. Organise and present findings to facilitate understanding and interpretation.
4. Avoid surprising primary stakeholders.
5. Prepare users to engage with and learn from 'negative' results.
6. Distinguish dissemination from use. (Patton 2008: 509)

Creating a draft report and sharing this with key stakeholders can ensure there are no surprises, but more than this, it can help in identifying any issues regarding clarity and presentation. Further, when done in a timely fashion, a draft report can present opportunities to reflect on and improve the inclusion of stakeholders' voices. These reports provide a useful means of engaging stakeholders in the review of findings and can facilitate a conversation between funders and evaluators in relation to expectations. O'Sullivan (2004: 142) argues 'Often sponsors are unaware of how evaluation findings will be represented. It is only when they see or hear about findings that they can make a determination about the level of acceptability.' She concurs with Patton, in asserting that the purpose of sharing a draft report is not to do with content, nor does it imply that evaluators should change results to keep the funder happy. The purpose is more to do with how knowledge is communicated and matching expectations in terms of format.

A good report is often seen as one that explicitly links the evaluation findings with the interests of the stakeholders (Gibson and Brown 2009). When writing up a report based mainly on qualitative data, as is often the case with small-scale participatory evaluations, a balance needs to be struck between the use of direct quotation (the words of the participants) and the summarisation and analysis of the data. There is a need to 'keep it real' in order to enable the reader to develop a sense of what has happened at a personal level. The aim is to connect the reader with the project participants. Essentially, an evaluation report needs to be both readable and convincing.

Green and South (2006) make an interesting point when they state that while large-scale and publically-funded evaluations see wider dissemination as an integral part of their dissemination strategy, small-scale evaluation projects often either overlook or underestimate the value and relevance of their work to others. They argue that 'many potentially useful evaluation reports on interventions carried out under everyday circumstances and in the real world, remain lost in the so-called 'grey literature' (Green and South 2006: 155). This is certainly true of youth and community work evaluations in the past, and has resulted in the perception amongst policy-makers, leaders and practitioners that there is no available knowledge base 'out there'. Small-scale projects are well placed to generate knowledge about programme implementation and the causal pathways of change. As such, reports should focus on communicating this knowledge rather than on whether an intervention works or not. Green and South (2006) present a useful template for reporting small-scale evaluations (see Table 12.1).

Some report templates will include an executive summary. Usually, this includes similar content to the conclusion and recommendations section in the above template along with a summary account of the evaluation aims and methods. Executive summaries, placed at the beginning of the report, are aimed at those who have limited time and who are unlikely to read the full report. For this reason, therefore, they need to be brief (ideally no more than two pages), clear and precise.

Although the provision of recommendations is seen by many, particularly by funders, as an essential element of evaluation reports, there is no universal agreement within the evaluation community about this. Stake (2004) makes the point

TABLE 12.1 Template for reporting small-scale project evaluation (adapted from Green and South 2006: 156)

Section	Content
Introduction: project information	• background, aims and objectives and theory of change • main activities and resources • target population • context
Evaluation methods	• description of data collection methods, sampling and approach to analysis • limitations of the evaluation
Findings	• evidence about success • enabling factors and context • barriers
Discussion: key issues and lessons learned	• the project's achievements or lack thereof • the particular aspects of the mode of delivery or the context that contributed or restricted achievements • whether any groups benefited to a greater extent than others and why • the strengths and weaknesses of the project • the major challenges in rolling the project out further that may be of relevance to managers and commissioners • what should continue and what should change • good practice which could be transferred to other projects
Conclusion and recommendations	• summary of the key points • concise recommendations which have emerged from the findings

that recommendations tend to be informed by the evaluator's thoughtful speculation rather than being empirically based. He advises evaluators to carefully consider any recommendations they might offer in relation to how these may impact on the stakeholders. Alkin et al. (2006: 394) question whether the provision of recommendations is beyond the role of the evaluator: 'The worry that we have with highly specific recommendations concerns the extent to which the evaluator goes beyond areas of evaluation expertise and ventures in to a consultant role requiring specific program expertise.'

Where no specific expertise exists, the evaluator may consider offering more general recommendations framed as alternatives to be considered. In participatory evaluation, this problem is reduced by stakeholder involvement in the process of generating recommendations. Arguably, this involvement will increase the likelihood of any recommendations made being appropriate, achievable and realistic.

Other forms of sharing knowledge

In the context of participatory evaluation, dissemination of evaluation findings is often directed towards community learning. Community learning is achieved through collaborative dialogue based on the data and supports the co-construction of knowledge and the development of social change strategies (Groundwater-Smith, Dockett and Bottrell 2015). It follows, therefore, that sharing knowledge in this context is likely to include a range of participatory activities that provide opportunities to develop further discussion. These activities may include oral presentations aimed at specific stakeholder groups, workshops for practitioners, media releases (print-based and web-based) or visual displays. Heath, Brooks, Cleaver and Ireland (2009) make a very good point when they highlight the fact that young people are rarely identified as members of the primary audience when planning for dissemination. The same can probably be said of community members. In order to communicate evaluation findings to young people and community members we need to think of alternatives to the written form and to consider more active dissemination processes.

Three alternative forms of disseminating findings, ethnodrama, speak-outs and imagery are briefly explained here, although many other forms exist.

Ethnodrama involves the evaluator and the participants using the evaluation data to develop a script that is primarily based on verbatim narrative. Importantly, the performance is accompanied by an opportunity for the audience to draw implications for themselves from the performance and to discuss these with each other and the cast (Mertens 2009). The use of ethnodrama as a means of dissemination is growing in popularity.

'Speak-outs' are another form of participatory dissemination. Originating in the 1960s, they continue to be a popular approach in community-based contexts. Speak-outs can take different forms but in essence, in the context of evaluation dissemination, they provide an interactive exhibition space. In this space, a variety of people have the opportunity to engage in an informal 'public meeting' about the findings of the evaluation (Sarkissian and Bunjamin-Mau 2009). Importantly, the evaluator and the participants co-facilitate the process.

The use of imagery provides a further means of both communicating knowledge and engaging audiences with the evaluation findings. Photographs, art work and video can be used to communicate the experiences of young people in compelling ways. These can be displayed or presented to audiences to promote discussion. Posters provide another means of effective way to communicate learning generated through evaluation and can be disseminated on a wider scale (Heath et al. 2009).

The value of using participatory forms of dissemination lies in the face-to-face encounter. The immediacy of contact enables an active engagement in dialogue between participants and audience. Additionally, the experience of 'presenting' information live supports the empowerment aspect of participatory evaluation and provides further learning opportunities for those involved.

However, it is important to take account of the challenges of taking a more participatory approach to dissemination. It can be a daunting task to present to an audience and this in itself may exclude some young people. There is a need to recognise that involving young people in the dissemination, especially when using verbatim narrative, threatens their anonymity. Publically 'owning' the message may also be an issue, as this may result in them being confronted by others about their interpretations. External evaluators tend to leave after the evaluation whereas community members remain. There is also a risk that when using creative forms of dissemination, the focus shifts towards the event and away from the message.

Meta-evaluation: sharing learning about evaluation

Participatory evaluations are shaped by those who use them and thus require a commitment to interrogate the assumptions, actions and outcomes arising from them. While attention is given to sharing evaluation findings, the sharing of learning about evaluation itself is often overlooked. It is important to review the process of evaluation as this can develop the evaluation capacity of those involved. Further, it can support sustainability and develop new understandings of 'what works well' in participatory evaluation. The process of evaluating our evaluation processes is termed meta-evaluation and involves attending to evaluation quality and developing evaluation knowledge, understanding and skills. Meta-evaluation can be understood both as an external study to authenticate the process and product of evaluation, and as a process of ongoing informal reviewing of the evaluation (Stake 2004).

An external meta-evaluation can provide credibility in a similar way that independent financial reports ensure credibility of profit reports (Patton 2008). However, small-scale evaluations will rarely have the resources for an independent meta-evaluation. For small-scale evaluations, the focus can justifiably be on developing a critically reflective examination of the evaluators' practice. For example, in Transformative Evaluation (see Chapter 6), meta-evaluation is used as an ongoing reviewing process. It is highlighted as a distinct stage in order to indicate its importance and value, and all participants engage in the process.

Participatory evaluation, by its very nature, involves a range of stakeholders, complex relationships and multiple perspectives. It is, therefore, essential that the process of meta-evaluation involves both reflection and reflexivity. Reflection is clearly an important part of the participatory evaluation process. Meta-evaluation uses reflection to raise questions about evaluative practice; did it have value or not? Did it work well? Did it do what we hoped it would? Does it need improving? How might it be developed further? These questions are of a technical nature, about our practical actions. Alongside this there is a need to be reflexive. Reflexivity can help us to increase our awareness of 'self' in the actions of conducting the evaluation, analysing data and constructing and representing outcomes. Through being reflexive, we develop awareness of our 'positionality', of how we are positioned by structural relations (for example, gender, race, class) and how the power implications of this impact on our view of the world. Meta-evaluation, when conducted as an ongoing process, can provide the structure and format for issues of power to be discussed throughout the evaluation, a key requirement if the commitment to participation is to be realised.

Reflection and reflexivity are often seen as something individuals do, and yet arguably, when used in collective spaces their potential to lead to transformational learning is greatly enhanced (Cooper 2014). Meta-evaluation can provide a context for ongoing collective conversations; however, taking a collective approach in itself, is not sufficient to ensure transformative learning (Ng and Tan 2009). The focus of these collective conversations needs to be balanced. Equal value needs to be placed on the technical aspects of the evaluation and the questioning of how values and power influence the quality of judgement, decision-making and practice wisdom. This enables a shift from problem-solving towards active collective reflection on the goals and values and issues of equity and social justice.

In summary, a clear and audience-appropriate means of communication needs to be developed to maximise the use of evaluation findings. The engagement of stakeholders in the dissemination of participatory evaluation findings will require additional time and resources. However, the benefits of their involvement are wide-ranging in terms of extending the reach and authenticity of message. Additionally, the involvement of stakeholders in this stage of the evaluation may support their longer-term engagement with the project. A key point is that the methods used to disseminate evaluation findings need to be fit for purpose. In the context of youth and community work, methods that are interactive and that make use of multi-media are likely to be useful, alongside the more formal reporting.

The sharing of knowledge generated through participatory evaluation is paramount if we wish to effectively communicate the purpose and value of youth and community work to a wider audience. The message will be stronger if it contains multiple voices. Clearly there are challenges that arise from a commitment to involve stakeholders in the process of dissemination, but these are outweighed by the many benefits. The 'dissemination of findings' stage is an ending, but importantly, for anyone using participatory evaluation, it is also a beginning. New understandings, ideas and challenges arise through the collaborative dialogues and build upon the evaluation findings. Energy and commitment is fostered through engagement, and together, these community learning outcomes can shape the project's future.

References

Alkin, M., Christie, C. and Rose, M. (2006) 'Communicating Evaluation', in I. Shaw, J. Greene and M. Mark (eds), *The Sage Handbook of Evaluation*, London: Sage Publications, pp. 384–403

Cooper, S. (2014) 'Putting Collective Reflective Dialogue at the Heart of the Evaluation Process', in *Reflective Practice: International and Multidisciplinary Perspectives*, Vol. 15(5), pp. 563–578

Gibson, W. and Brown, A. (2009) *Working with Qualitative Data*, London: Sage Publications

Green, J. and South, J. (2006) *Evaluation: Concepts and Approaches*, Maidenhead: Open University Press

Groundwater-Smith, S., Dockett, S. and Bottrell, D. (2015) *Participatory Research with Children and Young People*, London: Sage Publications

Heath, S., Brooks, R., Cleaver, E. and Ireland, E. (2009) *Researching Young People's Lives*, London: Sage Publications

Mertens, D. (2009) *Transformative Research and Evaluation*, London: Guilford Press

Ng, P. and Tan, C. (2009) 'Communities of Practice for Teachers: Sensemaking or Critical Reflective Learning?', in *Reflective Practice*, Vol. 10(1), pp. 37–44

O'Sullivan, R. (2004) *Practicing Evaluation: A Collaborative Approach*, London: Sage Publications

Patton, M. (2008) *Utilization-focused Evaluation* (4th ed.), London: Sage Publications

Sarkissian, W. and Bunjamin-Mau, W. (2009) *SpeakOut: The Step-by-Step Guide to SpeakOuts and Community Workshops*, Abingdon: Earthscan

Stake, R. (2004) *Standards-based & Responsive Evaluation*, London: Sage Publications

Stuart, K., Maynard, L. and Rouncefield, C. (2015) *Evaluation Practice for Projects with Young People*, London: Sage Publications

CONCLUSION

The thorny questions of 'what is youth work?' and 'what are youth work outcomes?' were raised in the Introduction to this book in order to establish the context for what follows. It was established that, whilst there is no universal definition of youth work across the world, there are a number of common features from which can be drawn a set of principles and values that apply across the board. These are that:

- the work must build from where young people are;
- the relationship between the young person and youth worker is central to the learning process;
- young people and youth workers are active partners in a learning process; and
- youth work engages with young people within their communities.

Evidently then, youth and community work is a dynamic and unpredictable process, and this presents challenges for anyone trying to evaluate the outcomes. The challenge is not at the practice level. Youth workers have always been able to identify the positive impact that their work has at an individual level, noticing the changes in young people's attitudes, behaviours and aspirations. The challenge arises at project, organisational and sector level, and the central argument of this book is that this is a consequence of the way in which outcomes and outcome measurement are conceived in contemporary society.

Part 1 of the book seeks to provide an in-depth and critical perspective of evaluation with the aim of enabling those involved in youth and community work to both recognise and challenge the dominant discourse. It is hoped that this will support workers, leaders and commissioners to recognise that change is possible and that, depending on our conceptualisation and enactment, evaluation can be:

- an inclusive process rather than an exclusive process;
- a liberating process rather than a controlling process;

- a defence rather than a threat; and
- a part of everyday practice rather than an imposition.

In Chapter 2 the political nature of evaluation is unpacked in order to dispel the myth that evaluation is a neutral process and to place the dominance of the quasi-experimental approach within the wider political context. This is not just an issue for youth and community work and there is value in recognising that all public services have been affected. For example, the quality of formal education is conceived in relation to grades achieved rather than a more holistic judgement that includes qualitative aspects such as student experience or their social and emotional learning.

The development of sets of standards may be seen by some to provide a transparent and neutral frame to apply judgement, yet it is argued in this book that these are in themselves political. The Bond Principles are introduced as an alternative – and arguably a more appropriate – set of principles. These are based on values that align well with youth and community work, for example, justice, solidarity, diversity, collaboration and participation. It is hoped that these principles will provide a way forward for those looking to challenge the dominant discourse. Part 1 concludes with a chapter that illuminates the risks to youth work and to youth workers if we continue to accept and conduct evaluation processes that are entirely informed by a quasi-experimental approach.

Part 2 of the book introduces participatory evaluation and makes the case for the use of participatory approaches in evaluating youth and community work on the basis of congruence between values and principles. The benefits of using a participatory approach for evaluating youth and community work were presented. While a number of different participatory approaches to evaluation have been developed, they share some common principles. These are:

- *participation*: multiple perspectives, experiences and democratic inclusion are recognised and valued;
- *learning*: focus is placed on practical or action-orientated learning, and learning is seen as an individual and collective process;
- *negotiation*: fostering dialogue and deliberation is central and contributes to a sense of shared ownership; and
- *flexibility*: the continually evolving nature of 'working together' is accepted.

Participation itself is a complex concept. Chapter 4 aimed to provide an in-depth examination of what this means in the context of evaluation in youth and community work. A range of participatory evaluation approaches were presented in Chapters 5 and 6. These were explored in detail. Examples from practice were introduced with the aim of providing sufficient knowledge and understanding for workers, organisations and commissioners to consider their use in their own context. This part of the book concluded with a chapter that examines the learning potential of participatory forms of evaluation. Importantly, the focus was on learning that arises from doing evaluation (what Patton calls 'process use') as this is often neglected when considering evaluation design. The learning potential is a considerable strength of participatory evaluation and can be used to support anyone making a case for using a participatory approach.

In Part 3 the emphasis was on the practicalities of conducting participatory evaluation, and the various stages were presented. At each stage of the evaluation journey, whether that is preparing for the evaluation, deciding what data are required and how they might be generated and analysed, or how learning can be shared, there is a need to consider, appraise and select the most appropriate options for the context. It is hoped that this part of the book will provide assistance to the reader in making these decisions along with support in terms of justifying their choices. Being able to do this will be essential in terms of challenging the dominance of quasi-experimental approaches. It is hoped that it will also enable those engaged in evaluation to confidently use (and develop) participatory evaluation appropriate to their setting.

Visioning change

The rationale for this book was to address the fact that evidencing the difference that youth and community work makes to the lives of young people and communities has been challenging the profession for decades. It has been argued that while considerable attention has been paid to developing evaluation frameworks and tools to aid practitioners to meet this challenge, these advances are of a technical nature and have not addressed the issue of the dominance of one particular form of evaluation – the quasi-experimental. Undoubtedly, there is a need to develop our understanding of 'what works and how' and to more effectively articulate the value of youth and community work to policy makers, funders and the wider society. How this is achieved, however, is questionable. It has been argued in this book that we need to critically consider the ways in which our evaluative practices enable or disenable us to do this.

We need to think again about the process of evaluation; in particular, we need to consider alternative paradigms which are more akin to youth and community work. The participatory paradigm, with its emphasis on stakeholder involvement, is quite different to the experimental evaluation paradigm and arguably generates different kinds of 'evidence'. Yet there is a danger in privileging any one type of evaluation evidence or evaluation methodology. This book is not promoting a shift from one paradigmatic position to another – from quasi-experimental to participatory – but it does seek to make the case for plurality.

Youth work outcomes are diverse, many cannot be prescribed, and as such there is a need to develop evaluation strategies that can appropriately and sufficiently represent the full range of possible outcomes. There is also value in developing an understanding of how these different ways of generating different types of evidence can inform and support one another.

Evaluation is an essential aspect of professional practice, and yet, many youth and community workers have become disengaged with the process as a consequence of the incompatibility of the quasi-experimental approach with their practice. While this is understandable, it is of great concern in terms of the future of youth and community work. It is hoped that this book will support students, practitioners, leaders and commissioners to question the status quo, to reconceptualise evaluation, and to develop a more diverse approach to evaluation practice. Change begins with small steps, and can be driven from the grass roots.

INDEX

Page numbers in italics refer to figures. Page numbers in bold refer to tables.